SPECIAL DIET COOK

DIABETIC ENTERTAINING

Mouth-watering meals for the health conscious

Azmina Govindji and Jill Myers

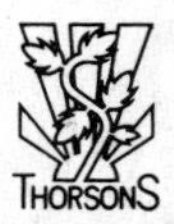

THORSONS PUBLISHING GROUP

Published in collaboration with
The British Diabetic Association
10 Queen Anne Street, London W1M 0BD

First published 1990

British Library Cataloguing in Publication Data

Govindji, Azmina
Diabetic entertaining: Mouth-watering meals for the health conscious.
1. Diabetics. Food — Recipes
I. Title II. Myers, Jill
641.5'6314

ISBN 0-7225-2134-0

Published by Thorsons Publishers Limited, Wellingborough, Northamptonshire NN8 2RQ, England

Typeset by Harper Phototypesetters Limited, Northampton, England
Printed in Great Britain by Bath Press, Bath, Avon

CONTENTS

FOREWORD

Food is a message of friendship, cooking a caring ritual, eating a way of celebrating. These deeply ingrained attitudes and feelings are common to all advanced human cultures.

But, those unfamiliar with diabetes may ask, what can the person with diabetes eat? Anything and everything, just what everyone else eats, what he or she has always eaten — but with a few important constraints. For those who need to inject insulin, timing and balancing the carbohydrate-containing foods are necessary to avoid the wide swings of glucose in the blood, upwards and downwards. Of course, the injections and the insulins can be timed and balanced too, to fit almost any kind of lifestyle. Less fatty food, replaced with more unrefined carbohydrate foods, will improve the cholesterol pattern in the blood and so protect the walls of the coronary and other arteries. For the overweight, general reduction of the daily food energy ('calorie') intake will encourage the body to use up its own fat stores, cause weight loss, improve the diabetes and health generally.

How does all this translate into the recipe you prepare, the menu you choose and the meal you eat? No foods are prohibited for the person with diabetes. It's a question of quantities and a matter of timing, all set within the pattern of personal preferences and cultural habit. It's a question of understanding — what are carbohydrates, what foods contain them, are all fats equally to be reduced, what is the energy ('calorie') content of a food? This information is just as important and just as interesting for the person without diabetes. We all need to understand more about the food we eat and to follow the same simple rules.

Diabetic Entertaining is designed to help with all these things. It provides ideas for dishes which make it easier to meet the constraints of diabetes but at the same time to enjoy the creativity of cooking for yourself and your family. With this book to help, you can all enjoy the pleasures of healthy eating.

Harry Keen MD, FRCP
Professor of Human Metabolism,
Director, Diabetes Services, and
Physician, Guy's Hospital,
London.

INTRODUCTION

How can you be sure that Mushroom Croustades, Coq au Vin and Summer Pudding will be suitable for your guests who have diabetes? Will your health-conscious friends approve of a buffet table laden with Turkey and Rice Ring, Salmon Pâté and Hummus? Will the Tuna Plait for the picnic be appropriate for the little boy who has just developed diabetes, or his sister who has a weight problem?

With *Diabetic Entertaining*, your problems are now over.

This book will broaden your culinary horizons with a range of practical ideas for ways to incorporate healthy-eating guidelines into special meals. Catering for health-conscious guests or a person with diabetes need not be a nightmare on the eve of a big dinner party.

Healthy eating does not mean that hors d'oeuvres need to consist only of carrot sticks or that the serving dish is filled with lettuce leaves garnished with a mere dollop of ratatouille. You can now serve up a range of eye-catching, mouth-watering calorie-counted gourmet dishes, enjoying a feast on your plate that will still help you keep a watchful eye on your waistline.

What is diabetes?

Diabetes mellitus is a very common disorder; it affects about 2 per cent of the UK population, and over 30 million worldwide. In simple terms, it is a condition in which the body is unable to control the amount of sugar (glucose) in the blood. This is because the mechanism which converts sugar to energy no longer functions properly. In well-controlled diabetes, the blood glucose level is close to the normal range (4–7 mmols per litre), while values consistently below 10 mmols per litre are quite satisfactory. Large fluctuations in blood glucose levels can impair the control of diabetes. Treatment for diabetes is designed to keep blood glucose at satisfactory levels and to delay or prevent serious complications developing in later life.

Diet is the fundamental part of treatment, although medication in the form of tablets or insulin injections can be required. A person with diabetes should see a dietitian, particularly when first diagnosed, and regularly thereafter if possible. The dietitian will provide specific advice on the type of diet to follow, the amount of each food to eat and practical ways of implementing the dietary guidelines.

Eating sensibly

The 'diabetic diet' is not in any way a special diet; in fact it is recommended for anyone who wishes to follow a healthy eating plan. It is close to the diet suggested for the whole population by the National Advisory Committee on Nutrition Education (NACNE) Report of 1983, and by the DHSS Committee on Medical Aspects of Food Policy (COMA) Document.

The recommendations are, in brief:

1. Try to maintain your ideal body weight (see weight chart).
2. Eat regular meals.
3. Eat more high-fibre, high-carbohydrate foods such as wholemeal bread, beans, lentils, and fruit.
4. Cut down on sugary foods and drinks.
5. Cut down on fats.
6. Eat less salt.
7. Keep alcohol consumption to a minimum.
8. Avoid special diabetic products.

Calories

The amount of energy you get from food is measured in calories and it is important to keep an eye on your calorie intake if you want to maintain your ideal weight. Being overweight can increase the risk of developing heart disease and diabetes; in those with diabetes, obesity can cause a deterioration in control. Having regular meals and keeping your calorie intake fairly constant from day to day is good practice, whether you have diabetes or not. Chapter 5 gives some tips on how to lose weight.

Take a straight line across from your height (without shoes) and a line up from your weight (without clothes). Put a mark where the two lines meet.

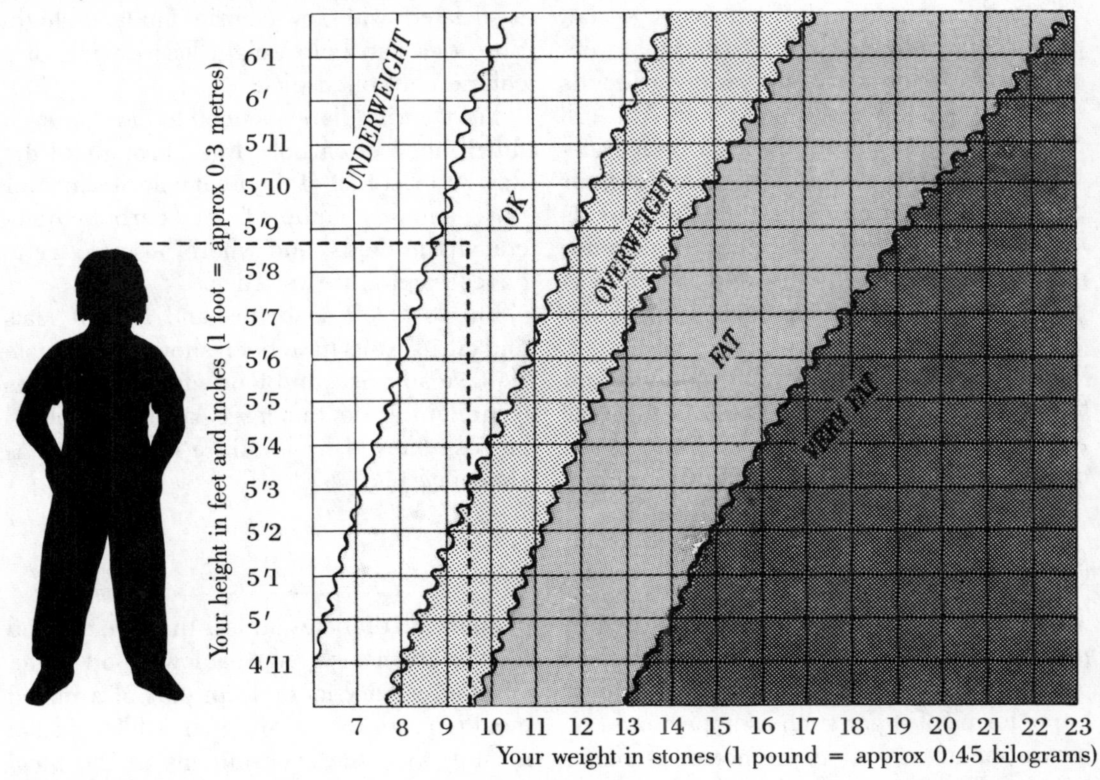

UNDERWEIGHT Maybe you need to eat a bit more. But go for well-balanced nutritious foods and don't just fill up on fatty and sugary foods. If you are *very* underweight, see your doctor about it.

OK You're eating the right *quantity* of food but you need to be sure that you're getting a healthy *balance* in your diet.

OVERWEIGHT You should try to lose weight.

FAT You need to lose weight.

VERY FAT You urgently need to lose weight. You would do well to see your doctor, who might refer you to a dietitian.

IF YOU NEED TO LOSE WEIGHT

Aim to lose 1 or 2 pounds a week until you get down to the 'OK' range. Go for fibre-rich foods and cut down on fat, sugar and alcohol. You'll need to take regular exercise too.

Fibre

All food is made up of nutrients — fat, protein, carbohydrate, fibre, vitamins, minerals, and water. Eating a variety of foods every day should ensure you have the full range of these nutrients. Carbohydrate-containing foods should form part of your main meal. High-fibre carbohydrate foods include wholemeal or granary bread, potatoes with their skins and other vegetables, brown rice, wholemeal pasta, wholegrain cereals, and fruits.

Fibre can help reduce constipation, and there also is some evidence to show that oats are particularly useful in lowering blood cholesterol levels. Being bulky and generally associated with low-calorie foods, a high-fibre diet can help weight loss as part of a calorie-controlled diet.

People with diabetes need to have an even distribution of carbohydrate throughout the day. At least half of the total calories in your diet should come from carbohydrate-containing foods, and where possible try to choose high-fibre varieties.

Pulses (such as beans and lentils), oats and citrus fruits have been shown to promote slow, steady rises in blood glucose, and this is preferable to the large swings in blood glucose caused by low-fibre foods (such as chocolate biscuits).

Sugar

Too much sugar can cause tooth decay, particularly if sweet foods and drinks are consumed at intervals throughout the day. Some forms of sugar such as honey and raw brown sugar are often promoted as being healthy. They do contain some vitamins and minerals but you would need to consume substantial amounts of them before you were to derive any significant nutritional benefits. It is far better to obtain those nutrients from other foods; and foods with a high sugar content are generally high in calories! Sweet foods are rapidly absorbed from the gut and can make blood sugar rise quickly — they should therefore be treated with caution by people with diabetes, unless they are needed in emergencies e.g. to treat low blood sugar.

When sugary foods form part of a mixed meal (e.g. an ice cream after a filled jacket potato), the other constituents in the meal (especially the fibre) allow the sugar to be absorbed at a slower rate. This means that the blood glucose does not rise as rapidly as it would if the ice cream was taken in isolation as a snack between meals. Most dietitians agree that a small piece of cake or other sweet food can be eaten occasionally at the end of a high-fibre meal.

It makes good sense for everyone, with or without diabetes, to limit their intake of sugary foods and drinks. The wide range of substitutes, not only artificial sweeteners (see page 13) but also low-sugar desserts, diet drinks, pure fruit spreads and so on, are of immense help when you want to have your cake and eat it!

Fats

Most experts advise that you should first try to reduce your total fat intake, and then substitute the saturated fat (e.g. meat and dairy products) with polyunsaturated sources (e.g. oily fish, polyunsaturated margarine, corn oil) wherever possible. Monounsaturated fats (e.g. olive oil) also make good replacements for saturated fats.

Eating too many fatty foods (particularly those containing saturated fat) has been shown to increase the level of cholesterol in the blood, which in turn increases the risk of developing coronary heart disease. Therefore, it is advisable to limit your fat consumption, especially if there is a family history of heart disease or if you have raised blood cholesterol levels. People with diabetes are at a greater risk of developing heart disease so, for you, reducing the amount of fat you eat is especially important. Weight for weight, pure fat has more than twice the calories of pure protein or carbohydrate, so cutting down on fats can also help you cut the calories.

Salt

High salt intakes have been linked with a greater risk of high blood pressure in some people. Try to get into the habit of using less salt in cooking and avoid adding salt at the table, and bear in mind that smoked meat and fish, cheese, sausages, yeast extract, corned beef, and some snack foods (e.g. crisps, nuts) all tend to be high in salt.

Alcohol

The Health Education Authority (H.E.A.) and the British Diabetic Association (B.D.A.) recommend that men should drink no more than three standard drinks a day, and women no more than two (women tend to be less able to tolerate alcohol than men).

1 standard drink (or 1 unit)	= ½ pint (285ml) of ordinary beer or lager	= a single measure of spirits (whisky, gin Bacardi vodka, etc.)	= a glass of wine (dry)	= a small glass of sherry (dry)	= a measure of vermouth or aperitif

All alcoholic drinks contain some alcohol and some sugar. Pure alcohol contains calories, in fact more calories than pure sugar. Alcoholic drinks provide none of the nutrients you need in a balanced diet. It is therefore better to keep your drinking well below the recommended level, particularly if you are overweight.

If you have diabetes, try to avoid drinking on an empty stomach. Alcohol in quantity causes low blood sugar (hypoglycaemia) which can be dangerous. Eating food with an alcoholic drink can reduce the risk of developing hypoglycaemia. Since this hypoglycaemic effect can last several hours, it is particularly important to have a snack (preferably one which is high in fibre) *after* you have been drinking alcohol.

Diabetic products

Special diabetic products are generally no lower in fat or calories than an equivalent non-diabetic food. They are often high in a sugar substitute called sorbitol (which can act as a laxative) and are expensive. As a small amount of cake or chocolate on an odd occasion after a high-fibre meal should not cause a rapid rise in blood sugar, there is little point in replacing these with a diabetic product. Look around instead for low-fat, low-sugar, low-calorie treats. Useful items to include instead of diabetic products are low-calorie squashes, diet drinks, reduced-sugar jam, wholemeal biscuits, crunchy cereal bars, fruits tinned in natural juice, and artificial sweeteners.

Sweeteners

There are two main groups of sugar substitutes: bulk (or nutritive) sweeteners and intense (or non-nutritive) sweeteners.

Bulk sweeteners

Examples of these are fructose (fruit sugar),

sorbitol, mannitol, isomalt, and xylitol. They are found in many diabetic products. Weight for weight, they provide around the same number of calories as ordinary sugar, so are not suitable for the overweight. They can be useful in baking (where creaming methods are used) and in preserving, but are not recommended for adding 'neat' to tea, coffee, cereals etc. because of their calorific value.

People with diabetes should take care not to consume more than a total of 25g (just under 1 oz) of bulk sweeteners per day. Larger quantities may have an adverse effect on the control of your diabetes and can also act as a laxative.

Numerous studies have shown that a moderate amount of sugar, when mixed with other foods, does not significantly affect the blood-sugar rise after a meal. In view of this, the B.D.A. has revised its recommendations. If you have diabetes, you can include up to a daily maximum of 25g (nearly an ounce) of sugar in home baking, provided you:

1. check with your dietitian first;
2. are not overweight;
3. are already keeping to a high-carbohydrate, high-fibre, low-fat diet;
4. are sure that the extra carbohydrate and calories can be fitted into your individual dietary allowance — the sugar should not be in addition to your normal diet, but part of it;
5. do not use the sugar in drinks, cereals, or in any instance where an artificial sweetener would suffice;
6. use the sugar in baking only where volume is required e.g. cakes, scones;
7. ensure that the other ingredients used in baking are high in fibre and low in fat;
8. do not eat the total allowance of 25g of sugar all at once, but spread it throughout the day.

Intense sweeteners

Examples of these are aspartame, acesulphame potassium (AcK), and saccharine. All are many times sweeter than sugar, and so only very small amounts are required. Supermarkets and chemists sell them under various brand names in granulated, tablet, and liquid forms, and they are also used in low-calorie sweet foods and diet drinks. Because of their lack of bulk, they cannot be used as a direct substitute for sugar in cooking.

As these sweeteners are virtually calorie-free, they are particularly suitable for people on a sugar-free or low-calorie diet. They can be sprinkled onto cereals or into custards, milk puddings or drinks.

Healthy eating tips

Fibre

- Choose high-fibre ingredients such as wholemeal flour for baking and cooking. Substituting half the white flour in a recipe with wholemeal flour is a good way to start.
- Try to include more peas, beans and lentils in your diet. In many dishes you can replace some of the meat with these pulses; this is cheaper, very nutritious and tasty!
- Using a pressure cooker saves time when cooking dried pulses — some don't even need soaking (check your pressure cooker instructions). Some varieties now are sold tinned and ready to use.
- Use brown rice, lentils and vegetables for nutritious salads, stir fries, and lentil burgers.

Sugar

- Choose intense sweeteners wherever possible or, better still, try to get into the habit of not using a sweetener at all. Use dried or fresh fruit when cooking — these can often provide enough sweetness without the need for sugar.
- Make use of your supermarket. Sugar-free yogurt, diet drinks, reduced-sugar jam, and tinned fruit in natural juice are only a small sample of what is available.
- If you don't like diet drinks, try making your own, using fizzy mineral water and unsweetened fruit juice.

Fat

- Low-fat dairy products are available in abundance. Take advantage of low-fat cheese, yogurt, milks, spreads, and half-fat cream substitute.
- Cut down on fatty foods such as chips, pastries, crisps, cakes, fatty meat, and meat products.
- Choose polyunsaturated fats (e.g. corn oil, sunflower oil, safflower oil, polyunsaturated margarine), or monounsaturated fats (e.g. olive oil, peanut oil) in preference to mixed vegetable oils, butter, margarine, or lard.
- Make sure your spreading-fat is soft when you use it — this makes it easier to spread so you use less.
- Get into the habit of draining off the fat which has settled on the top of cooked dishes. For example, if you are cooking mince, drain off all the liquid and allow this to cool in a refrigerator. When it has solidified, the fat can be removed from the surface and the tasty juices returned back to the meat. There is no need to add fat when browning meat.
- Choose fish, poultry, lean meat and

pulses instead of fatty meats. Buy low-fat varieties of sausages rather than the conventional types.

- Try not to add fat during cooking. Use the grill pan or the baking tray more often than the frying pan!
- When buying tinned fish, choose varieties which are tinned in brine and not in oil.
- Use skimmed milk in baking and in sauces, and semi-skimmed milk for drinks and cereals. These types contain less fat than ordinary milk but the same amount of calcium.
- Try using skimmed milk soft cheese or low-fat yogurt as a substitute for cream in sweet and savoury dishes.
- When using dried skimmed milk powder, choose one which has no added vegetable fat. Get into the habit of looking at the label!

About the recipes

This book contains a range of delicious and healthy recipes for that special occasion. All the ingredients used are in line with the recommendations already made — high in fibre, low in fat, and low in sugar. Low-fat spreads and polyunsaturated fats, low-fat dairy products, lean meats, and low-fat cooking practices have been used in compiling these recipes. High-fibre ingredients have been chosen wherever possible.

Small amounts of ordinary sugar have been included where its bulk is essential in some of the baked recipes (it is acceptable to include these foods occasionally as part of an overall healthy diet). If you do not wish to use ordinary table sugar you can replace it with a bulk sweetener such as fructose. Intense sweeteners have been used instead of sugar where volume is not required.

Where 'salt to taste' is indicated, try to use as little as possible. Be adventurous instead, and try enhancing the flavour of your cooked dishes with some of the wide range of herbs and spices available.

Each recipe has a designated total carbohydrate (CHO) and calorie (Cal) value which has been meticulously calculated using professional food composition tables. The former will be invaluable to people with diabetes who may be on a daily carbohydrate allowance; the latter will be of great help to those keeping an eye on their calories. In some recipes, the carbohydrate per portion works out to be around ¼ oz (5g) or less. This is an insignificant amount and it is more practical to exclude this contribution when calculating the carbohydrate value of the whole meal.

Note about conversions

As these recipes have all been tested using imperial measures, we have given the metric equivalent to the nearest 5g, rather than to the nearest 25g which is the convention in many cookery books. With some ingredients, such as tinned tomatoes, the conversion given on the tin may vary slightly.

Some ingredients, such as sachets of gelatine, are purchased in metric amounts, and here we give the imperial approximation.

For American readers

Please note the following differences between the American and British cookery terms:

British	American
1 teaspoon (5ml)	1¼ teaspoon
1 tablespoon (15ml)	1¼ tablespoon
1 pint (20 fl oz/570ml)	1¾ pints
8 fl oz (225ml)	1 cup
aubergine	eggplant
bicarbonate of soda	baking soda
butter beans	lima beans

British	American
chick-peas	garbanzos
coriander (fresh)	cilantro
cornflour	corn starch
courgettes	zucchini
ketchup	catsup
liquidize	blend
mangetout	snow peas
natural yogurt	plain yogurt
sieve	strain(er)
spring greens	collards
spring onion	scallion
tomato purée	tomato paste

HORS D'OEUVRES/ SOUPS/STARTERS

Hors d'oeuvres are essential for a sophisticated dinner party, where colourful 'finger foods' whet the appetite for larger quantities of cordon bleu cookery. Not only are they useful starters at the dinner table but they can also be served with pre-dinner drinks or used as one of the main dishes on a buffet table. If you are slimming you will find that many starters in this book are low in fat and calories — so filling up on these can help to cut down the inclination to indulge in what might be a calorific dessert. Many of these recipes are carbohydrate-free, so those with diabetes will still have the whole carbohydrate allowance for later courses.

French Onion Soup

Serves 4

1 tablespoon (15ml) corn or sunflower oil
1 lb (455g) onions, sliced into rings
1 clove garlic (optional)
2 tablespoons (30ml) wholemeal flour
2 pints (1.1 litres) beef stock
Sea salt and freshly ground black pepper

Total CHO Neg

Total Cals 280

1. Heat the oil in a large saucepan, add the onions, and garlic. Sweat over a gentle heat until transparent, taking care not to let the onions brown.
2. Stir in the flour, and cook for 2–3 minutes. Gradually stir in stock, and season to taste.
3. Bring to boil, cover, then simmer for 20 minutes.
4. Transfer to soup tureen and serve immediately.

Carrot and Tomato Soup

Serves 6–8

2 tablespoons (30ml) corn oil
2 onions, finely chopped
2 lb (905g) carrots, peeled and chopped
2×14 oz (2×400g) tins tomatoes
2 pints (1.1 litres) chicken or turkey stock
Finely grated rind and juice of 1 orange
Sea salt and freshly ground black pepper
Sprig of parsley

Total CHO 80g
Total Cals 620

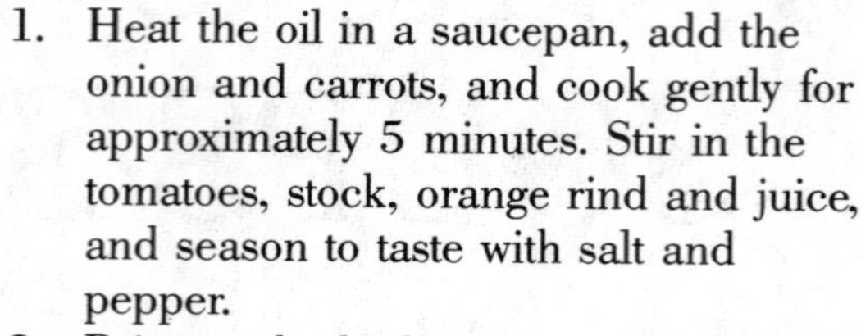

1. Heat the oil in a saucepan, add the onion and carrots, and cook gently for approximately 5 minutes. Stir in the tomatoes, stock, orange rind and juice, and season to taste with salt and pepper.
2. Bring to the boil, stirring, then lower the heat, half-cover with the lid, and simmer for 10–15 minutes until the carrots are tender.
3. Remove from the heat and leave to cool a little.
4. Purée in an electric blender or sieve to make a smooth purée. If the soup is too thick, stir in a little more stock or water. Taste and adjust seasoning.
5. Serve garnished with a sprig of parsley.

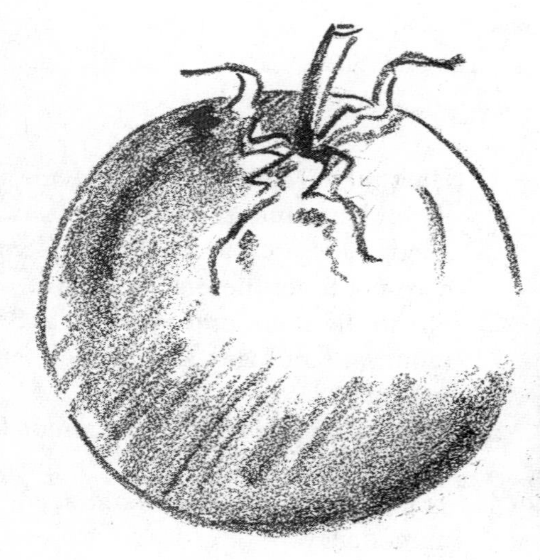

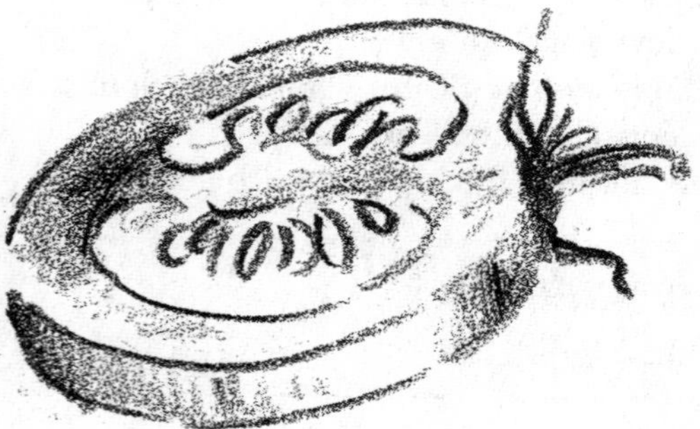

Gazpacho

Serves 4

1 lb (455g) ripe tomatoes, skinned, seeded and chopped
1 large Spanish onion, chopped
1 clove garlic, crushed
1 red pepper, seeded and chopped
Juice of 1 lemon
2 tablespoons (30ml) sunflower or olive oil
1–2 tablespoons (15–30ml) white wine vinegar
2 tablespoons (30ml) tomato purée
Sea salt and freshly ground black pepper
Parsley, chopped

1. Purée all the ingredients in an electric blender or food processor. Season to taste.
2. Put the soup in a tureen or serving bowl. Add enough water to make the soup a fairly runny consistency (a true Gazpacho is a thin soup).
3. Stand the tureen or bowl in a dish of ice cubes and chill in the refrigerator for 2–3 hours.
4. Just before serving, add a few ice cubes and chopped parsley.

Total CHO Neg

Total Cals 300

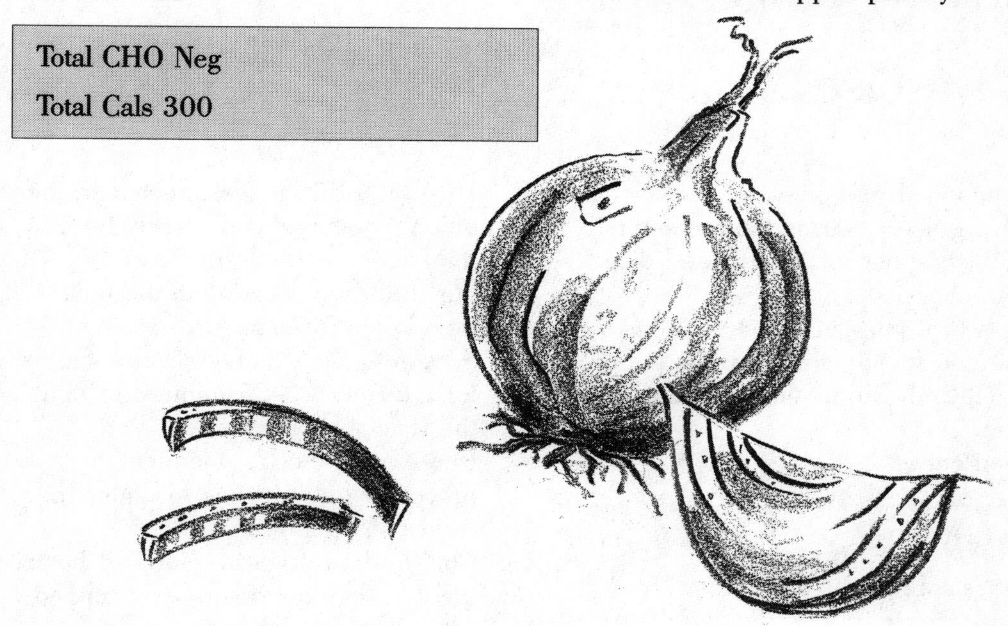

Watercress Soup

Serves 4–6

1 tablespoon (15ml) oil
1 onion, chopped
2 bunches watercress, washed and finely chopped (reserve a few sprigs for garnish)
1 medium potato, peeled and diced
½ pint (285ml) skimmed milk
1 pint (570ml) chicken stock
Sea salt and freshly ground black pepper

Total CHO 40g

Total Cals 380

1. Heat oil. Add vegetables and cook for 5 minutes.
2. Stir in the milk and stock, and bring to the boil. Add seasoning.
3. Lower the heat, cover, and simmer for approximately 30 minutes.
4. Purée the soup in an electric blender or food processor. Adjust seasoning.
5. Before serving, float a few leaves of watercress on the surface.

Vichyssoise

Serves 4–6

1 tablespoon (15ml) oil
1 lb (455g) leeks, washed and chopped
12 oz (340g) potatoes, peeled and diced
1 onion, chopped
1½ pints (850ml) chicken stock
Sea salt and freshly ground white pepper
5 fl oz (142ml) carton single or half-fat cream
Chopped chives

Total CHO 80g

Total Cals 520

1. Heat oil. Add the leeks, potatoes, and onion, cover and cook gently for 5 minutes.
2. Stir in the stock, bring to the boil, then lower the heat.
3. Season to taste, half-cover and simmer for a further 20–25 minutes or until the vegetables are tender.
4. Purée in an electric blender or processor until the soup is smooth. Adjust seasoning.
5. Chill in the refrigerator for 2–3 hours.
6. Swirl in the cream and serve topped with chopped chives.

Mushroom Soup

Serves 4–6

2 tablespoons (30ml) corn or sunflower oil
1 onion, chopped
1 lb (455g) mushrooms, cleaned and chopped
1 tablespoon (15ml) wholemeal flour
2 pints (1.1 litres) chicken stock
Sea salt and freshly ground black pepper
Pinch of grated nutmeg
1 bay leaf
Fresh parsley, chopped
Swirl of single or half-fat cream

Total CHO 10g
Total Cals 380

1. Heat the oil in a large pan. Add the onion and mushrooms, cover and cook gently for 5 minutes.
2. Stir in the flour and continue cooking for a further 2 minutes, stirring constantly.
3. Gradually add the chicken stock and bring to the boil, stirring. Add the seasoning.
4. Lower the heat, half-cover, and simmer gently for a further 20 minutes.
5. Purée the soup in an electric blender. Adjust seasoning.
6. Before serving, sprinkle with parsley and add a swirl of cream.

Tuna Dip

Serves 4

1×7 oz (200g) tin tuna in brine, drained
4 tablespoons (60ml) low-calorie mayonnaise
3 tablespoons (45ml) low-fat natural yogurt
1 tablespoon (15ml) tomato ketchup
1 tablespoon (15ml) lemon juice
1 teaspoon (5ml) Worcestershire sauce
2 spring onions, chopped
Freshly ground black pepper
Selection of vegetable crudités

1. Place the ingredients in a bowl and mix well. Season with freshly ground black pepper.
2. Place in a serving dish and chill before serving with a selection of crudités.

Total CHO Neg
Total Cals 430

Salmon Pâté

Serves 6

- 1×7½ oz (213g) tin red or pink salmon or tuna in brine
- 4 oz (115g) quark or skimmed-milk cheese
- Juice of ½ lemon
- 2 tablespoons (30ml) low-fat natural yogurt (optional)
- Freshly ground black pepper
- Lemon slices
- Sprig fresh parsley
- Melba toast

1. Place the salmon, cheese, lemon juice and yogurt into a bowl, and work until smooth. Season with freshly ground black pepper.
2. Smooth into six individual dishes or one large serving dish and chill before serving garnished with lemon slices and a sprig of parsley. Serve with melba toast.

Total CHO Neg

Total Cals 420

Chicken Liver Pâté

Serves 4–6

- 1 oz (30g) low-fat spread
- 1 tablespoon (15ml) oil
- 1 onion, chopped
- 1 clove garlic, crushed
- 12 oz (340g) chicken livers
- Sea salt and freshly ground black pepper
- Grated nutmeg
- 1 tablespoon (15ml) dry sherry
- Lemon slices
- Bay leaf

1. Place the low-fat spread, oil, onion and garlic in a bowl, and microwave on high for 3 minutes, stirring once.
2. Add the chicken livers and seasonings. Continue cooking for 4 minutes on high, stirring twice. Cool.
3. Liquidize until smooth and stir in the sherry. Place in a dish and smooth the top. Garnish the top with lemon slices and a bay leaf.
4. Chill before serving.

Total CHO Neg

Total Cals 700

Canapés

These are bite-sized and attractive to look at.

Suitable bases:
Small squares of wholemeal bread or toast
Wholemeal biscuits or crackers
Mini oatcakes

Toppings to spread on the base try:
Skimmed-milk cheese
Low-fat spread
Reduced-calorie mayonnaise
Pâtés

Decoration
Left-over bits and pieces e.g. chicken, cooked ham, or tinned fish
or Thin slivers of smoked salmon or anchovies
Thin slices of tomato
Sliced olives
Cocktail onions
Sliced gherkins

Salmon Pâté with Dill Mayonnaise

Makes 6

2×7½ oz (213g) tins red salmon, drained and flaked
1 teaspoon (5ml) lemon juice
4 oz (115g) skimmed-milk cheese
2 tablespoons (30ml) whipping cream
1 oz (30g) fresh wholemeal breadcrumbs
Sea salt and freshly ground black pepper

For the dill mayonnaise:

4 tablespoons (60ml) reduced-calorie mayonnaise
1–2 tablespoons (15–30ml) low-fat natural yogurt
2 sprigs fresh dill, chopped

Total CHO 10g
Total Cals 1330

1. Mix the flaked salmon with the lemon juice. Beat the cheese and cream together, then stir in the salmon mixture and breadcrumbs.
2. Season to taste. Divide the pâté mixture between 6 small ramekins.
3. Cover and chill in the refrigerator for at least an hour or preferably overnight.
4. Meanwhile, mix the mayonnaise with the yogurt and add the dill. Season well to taste.
5. Just before serving, turn each salmon pâté out onto a small serving plate and add a spoonful of dill mayonnaise, or serve the mayonnaise separately.

Hummus

Serves 4

1×14 oz (400g) tin chick-peas, drained
Juice of 1–2 lemons
4 tablespoons (60ml) tahini paste
1–2 cloves garlic, crushed
Sea salt and freshly ground black pepper
Paprika
Fresh coriander leaves

Total CHO 40g

Total Cals 470

1. Place the chick-peas and lemon juice in a food processor or blender. Process until smooth.
2. Add the tahini paste and garlic, and season to taste. Process to a smooth creamy paste.
3. Garnish with a sprinkling of paprika and roughly chopped fresh coriander leaves.

Cucumber and Prawn Starter

Serves 6–8

1 large cucumber
3 tablespoons (45ml) reduced-calorie mayonnaise
1 tablespoon (15ml) tomato ketchup
Dash Worcestershire sauce
1 tablespoon (15ml) dry sherry
Sea salt and freshly ground black pepper
6 oz (170g) frozen peeled prawns, defrosted
Paprika for sprinkling

Total CHO Neg

Total Cals 310

1. Chop the stalk end from the cucumber. Slice the cucumber into eight equal rings and hollow out the centres with a teaspoon to make a cup shape.
2. Mix together in a bowl the mayonnaise, tomato ketchup, Worcestershire sauce, sherry and prawns. Season to taste.
3. Spoon this mixture into the cucumber cups.
4. Sprinkle with paprika and chill for 30 minutes before serving.

Mushroom Croustades

Makes 8

4 small slices of sliced bread, crusts removed
½ oz (15g) low-fat spread
4 oz (115g) button mushrooms, sliced
4 rashers of bacon, chopped small
1 small onion, finely chopped
1 clove of garlic, crushed
1 tablespoon (15ml) parsley, chopped

Total CHO 40g

Total Cals 660

1. Cut each slice of bread in half. Spread both sides of bread with low-fat spread and press down in patty or jam tart tins, to form cup shapes. Bake the cups in the tins in a 400°F/200°C (Gas Mark 6) oven for 5–7 minutes until crisp and golden brown.
2. Meanwhile, lightly fry mushrooms, bacon, onion and garlic until onion is soft. Remove from heat.
3. Fill cooked cases and sprinkle with the parsley.
4. Reheat in the oven for 1–2 minutes until warm. Serve immediately.

Apple and Kiwi Salad

Serves 4

2 red apples, cored and sliced
2 kiwi fruit, peeled and sliced
Lemon juice
1 oz (30g) sunflower seeds
Lettuce or salad leaves

Total CHO 30g

Total Cals 320

1. Toss the sliced apples in a bowl with lemon juice to prevent discolouration. Add kiwi fruit and toss.
2. Arrange a bed of lettuce or salad leaves on 4 individual plates and spoon the fruit mixture on top.
3. Sprinkle with sunflower seeds. Serve immediately.

Stuffed Eggs

Makes 24 (halves)

12 eggs, hard-boiled
¼ pint (140ml) reduced-calorie mayonnaise
1 tablespoon (15ml) curry powder
Sea salt and freshly ground black pepper
10–12 stuffed olives, sliced

Total CHO Neg
Total Cals 1430

1. Halve the eggs lengthwise. Scoop the egg yolks into a bowl and mash with a fork. Mix with the mayonnaise, curry powder and seasoning to taste.
2. Pipe or spoon the mixture into the reserved egg whites.
3. Garnish each half with a slice of stuffed olive. Chill before serving.

Fruit in Vinaigrette

Serves 4–6

1 paw-paw, peeled, seeded and cut into chunks
1 pear, peeled, cored, and cut into chunks
1 grapefruit, peeled and segmented
½ honeydew melon, peeled and cut into chunks
4 tablespoons (60ml) vinaigrette dressing
A few sprigs fresh mint

1. Mix the fruits together in a bowl. Pour over the dressing. Toss well.
2. Chill in refrigerator before serving. Garnish with fresh mint to serve.

Total CHO 80g
Total Cals 360

Avocado with Tangy Dressing

Serves 4

2 ripe avocados, peeled, halved, and stoned

For the dressing:

5 fl oz (142ml) carton soured cream or low-fat natural yogurt
1 tablespoon (15ml) white wine vinegar
1 tablespoon (15ml) olive oil
½ teaspoon (2.5ml) mustard powder
Sea salt and freshly ground black pepper to taste

Total CHO Neg
Total Cals 1050

1. Cut the avocado halves from the wide base at equal intervals almost to the top and fan out on 4 individual serving plates.
2. Mix the dressing ingredients together. Pour a little around the avocados.
3. Serve the remaining dressing separately. Serve immediately.

or

1. Cut the avocados in half (leaving the skin on) and remove the stone.
2. Fill the cavity with some dressing and serve remaining dressing separately. Serve immediately.

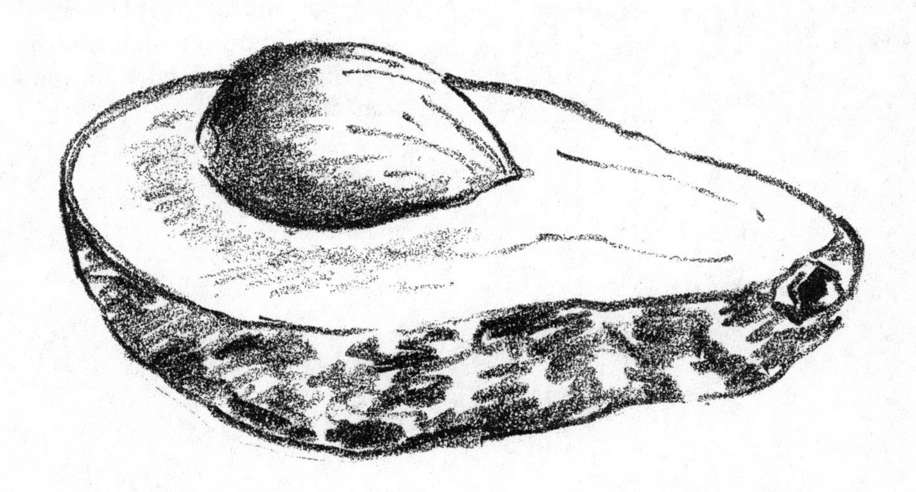

Courgettes Maison

Serves 4

8 small or 4 medium courgettes
1 tablespoon (15ml) corn oil
4 medium tomatoes, skinned and chopped
1 onion, finely chopped
1 clove garlic, crushed
4 oz (115g) prawns
1 teaspoon (5ml) paprika

For the mornay sauce:

1 oz (30g) low-fat spread
1 oz (30g) wholemeal flour
½ pint (285ml) skimmed milk
2 oz (55g) low-fat Cheddar cheese, grated
Extra grated cheese for topping
Paprika

Total CHO 60g

Total Cals 770

1. Wash and trim the courgettes. Cook in salted water for 5 minutes. Drain and refresh in cold water.
2. Remove a slice lengthways from each courgette and scoop out the insides with a teaspoon. Chop up the flesh.
3. Heat the oil and add courgette flesh, tomatoes, onion and garlic. Cook briskly for 3–4 minutes then add the prawns and paprika. Spoon the filling inside the courgette cases and place in an ovenproof dish.
4. Place all the ingredients for the sauce in a pan and heat until thick, stirring continuously. Pour over courgettes and sprinkle with the extra cheese.
5. Bake at 450°F/230°C (Gas Mark 8) for 15 minutes or until brown.
6. Serve hot, sprinkled with a little paprika.

FISH DISHES

Fish can be made into nutritious and delicious low-calorie meals which do not have to take all day to prepare. It is a valuable source of the B vitamins and of minerals such as calcium. There are two main categories of fish: oily fish such as herring and mackerel, and white fish such as cod and halibut. Fish oils are rich in vitamins A and D and essential fatty acids. A particular type of fat (called omega-3 fatty acid) found in oily fish has been shown to protect against heart disease. All this, and it tastes good too!

Seafood Sauce

Serves 2

1 medium onion, chopped
1 small green pepper, sliced
1×8 oz (225g) tin of tomatoes
2 oz (55g) mushrooms, sliced
1×4 oz (100g) tin tuna in brine, drained
1×4 oz (100g) tin prawns in brine, drained
1 oz (30g) unsalted cashew halves

1. Place all the vegetables in a pan. Bring to the boil and simmer gently for approximately 15 minutes or until onion and pepper are tender.
2. Stir in the tuna, prawns and cashew nuts. Cook for a further 5 minutes. Serve immediately.

Total CHO Neg

Total Cals 400

Chinese Fish with Ginger

Serves 2–4

1 lb (455g) haddock, cut into 1-inch (2.5cm) squares
Pinch of sea salt
½ teaspoon (2.5ml) ground ginger
1 tablespoon (15ml) cornflour
1-inch (2.5cm) piece fresh root ginger, peeled and finely chopped
4 spring onions, chopped
1 tablespoon (15ml) red wine vinegar
2 tablespoons (30ml) dry sherry
2 tablespoons (30ml) soya sauce
3 tablespoons (45ml) unsweetened orange juice
3 tablespoons (45ml) corn or sunflower oil

1. Mix together the salt, ground ginger and cornflour. Toss the fish in the mixture and set aside.
2. Mix together half the root ginger and spring onions, and add the vinegar, sherry, soya sauce and orange juice. Reserve.
3. Heat the oil, add the remaining root ginger and spring onions and stir-fry for 1 minute. Add the fish and fry for 3 minutes.
4. Pour on the vinegar mixture and bring to simmer for 3 minutes.
5. Serve immediately.

Total CHO 20g
Total Cals 800

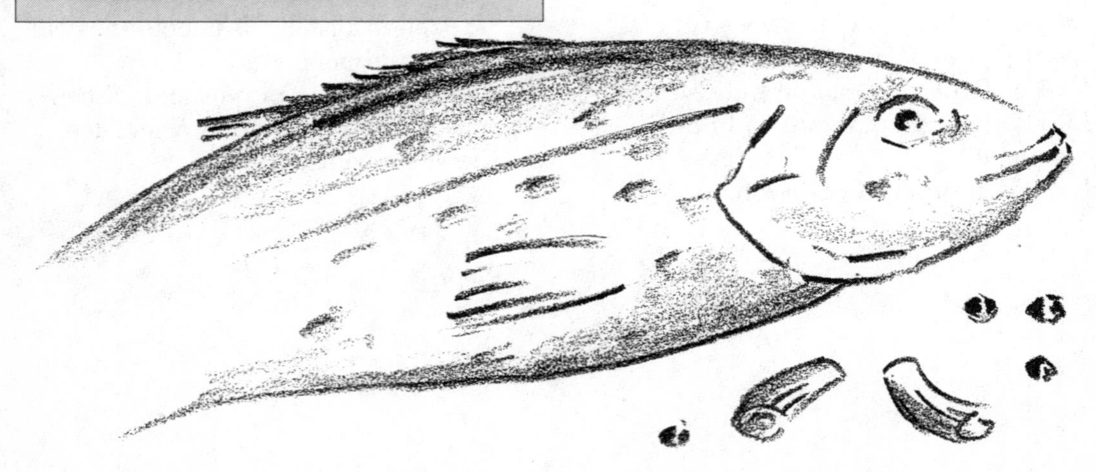

Stir-fried Prawns and Broccoli

Serves 4

1 dessertspoon (12ml) corn or sunflower oil
¼ teaspoon (1.25ml) cumin seeds
2 cloves garlic, crushed
1 bunch spring onions, chopped
6 oz (170g) broccoli heads, broken into small florets
5 oz (140g) prawns
1 dessertspoon (12ml) light soya sauce
¼ teaspoon (1.25ml) lemon juice

1. Heat oil in a wok or large pan. Add cumin seeds and garlic and cook for a few seconds.
2. Add onion and broccoli. Cook for 1–2 minutes before adding the prawns, soya sauce and lemon juice.
3. Serve immediately.

Total CHO Neg

Total Cals 280

Seafood Salad with Thousand Island Dressing

Serves 4–6

1 tablespoon (15ml) stuffed olives, finely chopped
1 small onion, finely chopped
1 size 3 egg, hard-boiled, chopped
1 small green pepper, deseeded and chopped
1 teaspoon (5ml) fresh parsley, chopped
1 teaspoon (5ml) tomato purée
Sea salt and freshly ground black pepper
¼pt (140ml) reduced-calorie mayonnaise
3 oz (85g) pasta shells, cooked
1×4oz (99g) tin salmon, drained and flaked
½ tub mustard and cress
4 oz (115g) peeled prawns

1. Mix together the olives, onion, egg, pepper, parsley, tomato purée, salt, pepper and mayonnaise. Chill.
2. Meanwhile, fold the pasta, salmon, mustard and cress and prawns together in a large bowl until thoroughly mixed. Pour over dressing and toss to coat.

Total CHO 50g

Total Cals 850

Trout with Lemon Stuffing

Serves 2

2 trout, gutted and thawed if frozen
1 oz (30g) wholemeal breadcrumbs
1 tablespoon (15ml) fresh parsley, chopped
1 tablespoon (15ml) fresh dill, chopped
1 small onion, peeled and chopped
1 stick celery, finely chopped
½ oz (15g) blanched almonds, chopped
Sea salt and freshly ground black pepper
2 lemons
2–3 sprigs of fresh dill

Total CHO 10g
Total Cals 600

1. Rinse the trout's insides. Place breadcrumbs, parsley, dill, onion, celery and almonds in a bowl. Add the finely grated zest and juice from one lemon. Season to taste.
2. Fill each fish cavity with this stuffing.
3. Place side by side in a lightly oiled baking dish. Slice half remaining lemon and reserve. Squeeze juice from other half over the fish.
4. Cover and bake at 375°F/190°C (Gas Mark 5) for 20–25 minutes. Uncover the fish after 10 minutes.
5. Arrange reserved lemon slices over top and garnish with dill. Serve hot.

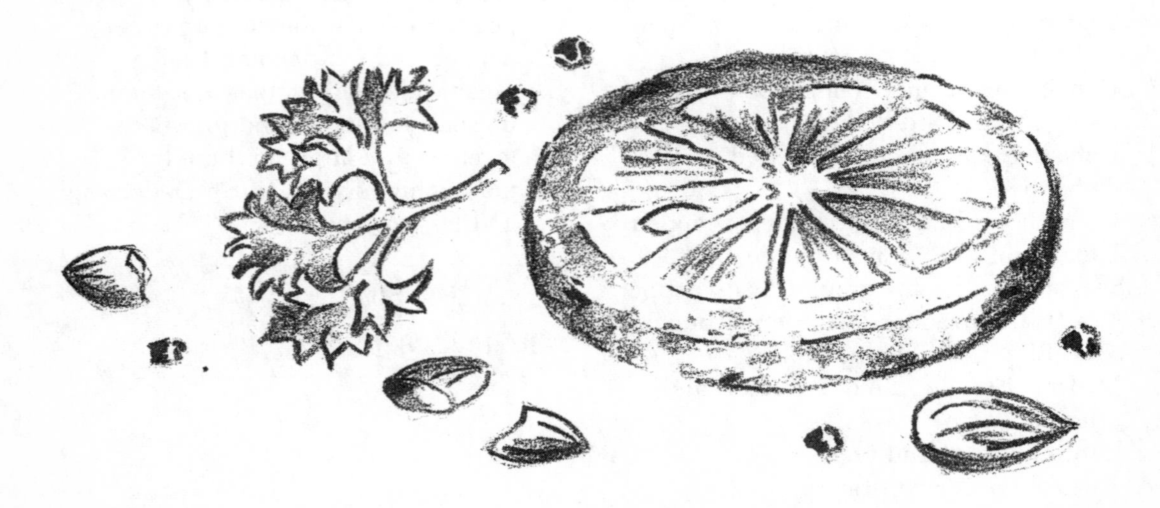

Haddock and Prawn Pie

Serves 4

12 oz (340g) haddock fillets
½ pint (285ml) skimmed milk
Sea salt and freshly ground black pepper
1 oz (30g) low-fat spread
1 onion, chopped
1 oz (30g) wholemeal flour
2 tablespoons (30ml) whipping cream
2 tablespoons (30ml) fresh parsley, chopped
1 tablespoon (15ml) lemon juice
4 oz (115g) prawns
1lb (455g) potatoes, peeled, cooked and mashed

Total CHO 120g

Total Cals 1070

1. Poach the haddock in the seasoned milk. Drain fish and reserve the liquid. Remove the skin from the fish and flake the flesh.
2. Melt the low-fat spread and lightly sauté the onions. Add flour, mix well. Add the milk and bring to the boil stirring continuously.
3. Adjust seasoning, stir in cream, parsley, lemon juice, prawns and flaked haddock. Mix well.
4. Pour into a serving dish and cover completely with the mashed potato. Bake in a 400°F/200°C (Gas Mark 6) oven for 20–25 minutes.
5. Serve immediately.

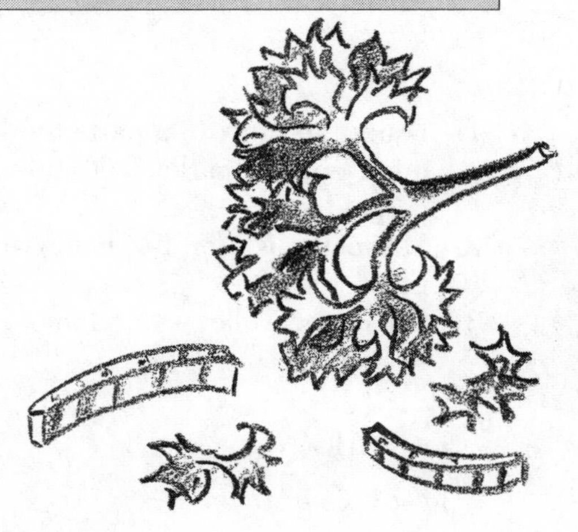

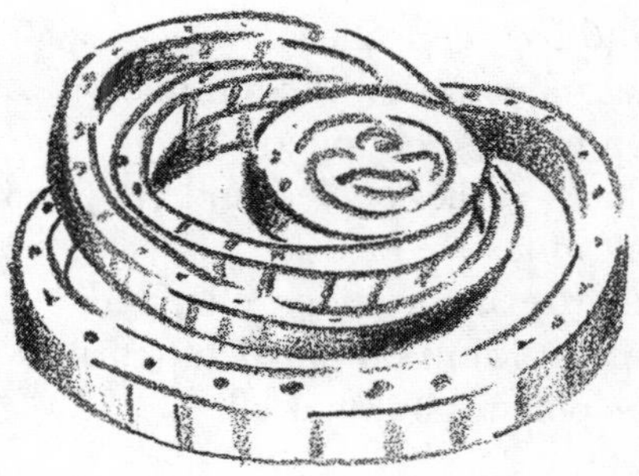

Orange and Lemon Stuffed Plaice

Serves 4

4 plaice fillets, skinned
1 orange
1 lemon
2 oz (55g) wholemeal breadcrumbs
1 egg, beaten
¼ pint (140ml) dry white wine or stock
Sea salt and freshly ground black pepper

Total CHO 30g

Total Cals 700

1. Lay the fillets on a clean non-wooden board.
2. Grate the rind from the orange and lemon. Peel the orange and remove the segments. Mix together the orange and lemon rind, orange segments, breadcrumbs and beaten egg.
3. Divide the mixture between the 4 fillets. Roll up the fillets and secure with a cocktail stick.
4. Place the fish in a shallow ovenproof dish and pour over the wine or stock. Season well. Cover and cook at 375°F/190°C (Gas Mark 5) for 30 minutes.
5. Serve immediately.

Masala Grilled Fish

Serves 3–4

1½ lb (680g) cod fillets
2 tablespoons (30ml) lemon juice
3 green chillies, chopped
4–6 cloves garlic, peeled and chopped
Sea salt to taste
1 bunch fresh coriander, chopped
1 teaspoon (5ml) oil per fillet (corn or other polyunsaturated oil)

1. Pound and mix to a paste the lemon juice, chillies, garlic, salt and coriander.
2. Marinade fish for 1–2 hours in this paste.
3. Brush each fillet with oil and grill until cooked.

Total CHO Neg

Total Cals 560

Prawn Curry

Serves 2–3

2 tablespoons (30ml) polyunsaturated oil
1 onion, chopped
3 cloves garlic, peeled and crushed
1 lb (455g) peeled prawns
2 teaspoons (10ml) garam masala powder
1 teaspoon (5ml) chilli powder
½ teaspoon (2.5ml) ground turmeric
Sea salt
¼ pint (140ml) water
Coriander leaves, chopped
2 tomatoes, sliced
Twist of lemon

1. Heat the oil in a pan and gently fry the onion and garlic until tender. Add the prawns and continue frying until dry.
2. Add the garam masala, chilli powder and turmeric, stir well and fry for 30 seconds. Add salt and the water.
3. Cover and cook gently for 10–15 minutes until dry.
4. Garnish with the coriander leaves and arrange the tomato slices and lemon on top.
5. Serve as a side dish with rice or bread.

Total CHO Neg

Total Cals 640

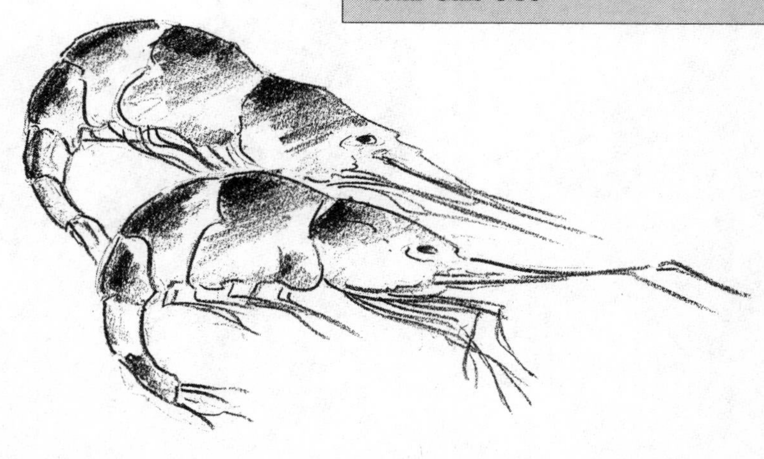

Tuna and Chick-pea Salad

Serves 4

1×15 oz (400g) tin chick-peas, drained
7 oz (200g) tin tuna in brine, drained and flaked
1 green pepper, seeded and sliced
2 tomatoes, chopped
1 small onion, sliced
8 black olives, stoned and halved (optional)
3 tablespoons (45ml) reduced-calorie mayonnaise
Sea salt and freshly ground black pepper

1. Put the chick-peas, tuna, green pepper, tomatoes, onion and black olives in a bowl. Mix well.
2. Fold in the mayonnaise and season to taste.
3. Chill lightly before serving.

Total CHO 60g

Total Cals 670

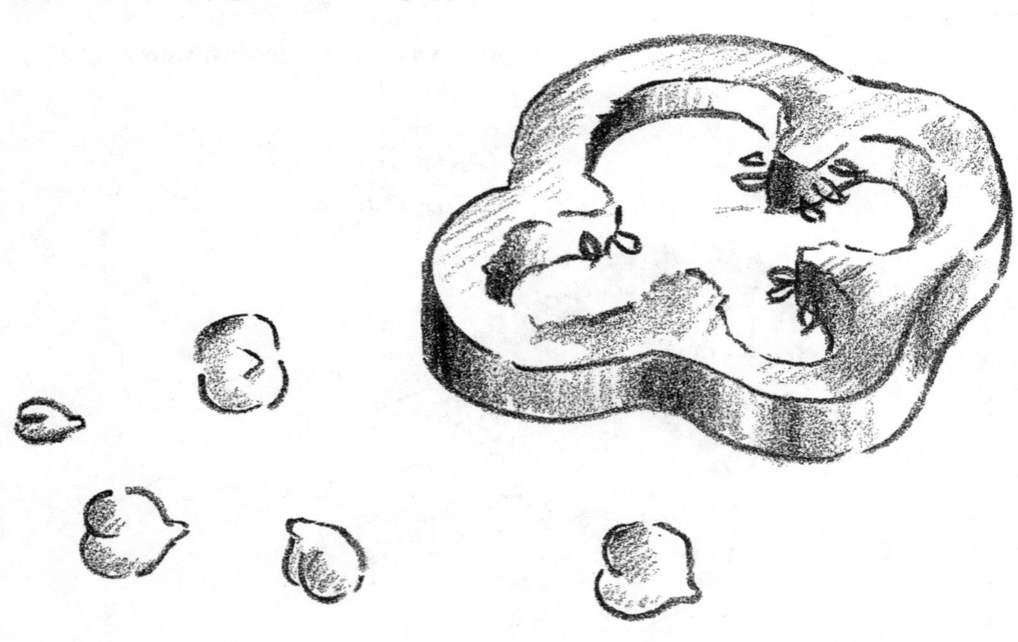

Tuna Plait

Serves 4

1×7 oz (200g) tin tuna in brine, drained
4 oz (115g) curd cheese and chives
4 oz (115g) sweet corn
2 tablespoons (30ml) skimmed milk
Sea salt and freshly ground black pepper
1×12 oz (340g) packet frozen wholemeal puff pastry, defrosted
Beaten egg to glaze

Total CHO 150g

Total Cals 1840

1. Place the tuna, cheese and sweet corn in a bowl. Mix well. Add the milk and season to taste.
2. On a floured surface, roll out the pastry to a rectangle 10 in.×15 in. (25cm×40cm). Place on a baking sheet. Mark into three sections lengthways.
3. Spoon the filling down the centre, to within 1 in. (2.5cm) of the short edges. Cut the pastry down each side of the filling into diagonal strips ½ in. (1cm) apart. Brush with beaten egg. Take one strip from each side of the pastry and cross them over the fish. Continue folding over the pastry strips from alternate sides of the filling to give a plaited effect.
4. Dampen top and bottom ends of the plait and fold over to seal. Brush all over with beaten egg and bake at 400°F/200°C (Gas Mark 6) for about 40–45 minutes, until crisp and golden.

MEAT AND POULTRY

Red meat and liver are rich sources of iron, protein and fat-soluble vitamins. Trimming the fat from fatty cuts of meat, or choosing the leaner cuts, reduces the amount of saturated fat present. Remember there is also hidden fat within the fibres of the meat — some of this can be drained off after cooking. The white meat of chicken and turkey is low in fat, particularly if the skin is removed. Meat can be the core of a meal and the traditional Sunday roast is still for many the highlight of the weekend. The recipes that follow will provide you with some alternative and exciting ways of dishing up a meaty meal that can be healthy.

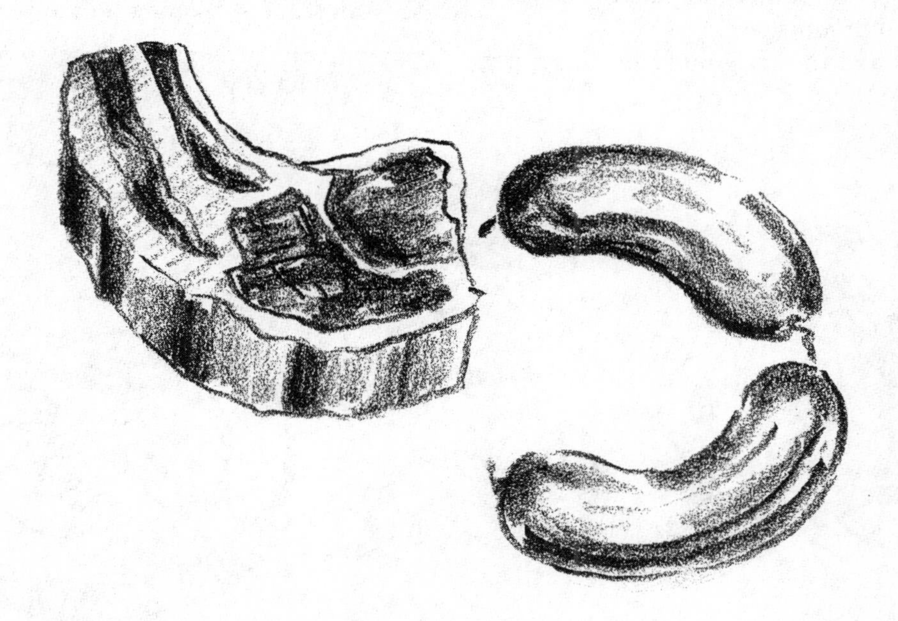

Hungarian Pork Goulash

Serves 4

1 tablespoon (15ml) sunflower oil
1½/2 lb (675g) pork, cut into 1-inch (2.5cm) cubes
2 onions, chopped
1 clove garlic, crushed
1 red pepper, sliced
1 green pepper, sliced
1–2 tablespoons (15–30 ml) paprika
1 tablespoon (15ml) wholemeal flour
1 tablespoon (15ml) tomato purée
1×14oz (400g) tin tomatoes
½–1 teaspoon (2.5–5ml) caraway seeds
½ pint (285ml) stock
Sea salt and freshly ground black pepper

1. Heat oil and fry the pork over a high heat to seal the meat. Add the onion and garlic and stir-fry 1–2 minutes. Add the peppers and cook for a further 1–2 minutes. Add the paprika, flour, tomato purée, tomatoes, caraway seeds and stock.
2. Cook for approximately 10 minutes. Season to taste.
3. Place the ingredients in a casserole dish and cook for 1½–2 hours at 300°F/150°C (Gas Mark 2).
4. Adjust the seasoning before serving.

Total CHO 10g
Total Cals 1730

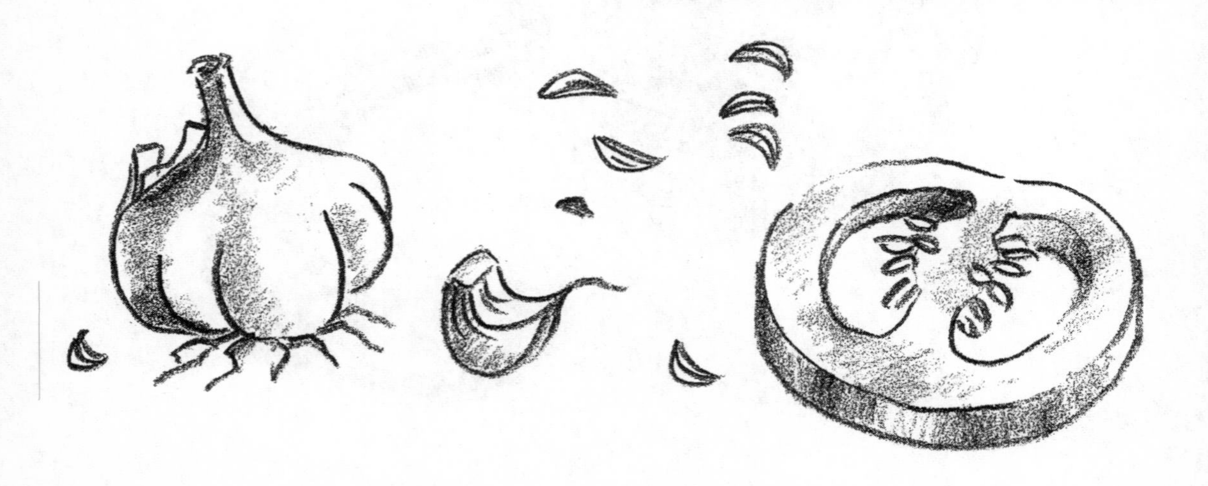

Pork Satay with Peanut Sauce

Makes 8

For the marinade:

1 clove garlic, crushed
1 teaspoon (5ml) chilli sauce
2 tablespoons (30ml) light soy sauce
2 tablespoons (30ml) dry sherry
2 tablespoons sunflower oil
1 teaspoon (5ml) ground ginger
1 lb (455g) pork fillet, cut into small cubes

For the peanut sauce:

2 oz (55g) no-added-sugar crunchy peanut butter
½ teaspoon (2.5ml) hot chilli powder
A few drops lemon juice
3 fl oz (90ml) water
½ oz (15g) creamed coconut

1. Mix all marinade ingredients together in a bowl. Leave meat to marinade for at least 2 hours but preferably overnight in the refrigerator.
2. Place all the ingredients for the sauce in a saucepan. Gradually bring to the boil, stirring all the time, until creamed coconut has melted and formed a sauce. The sauce should be a thick pouring consistency.
3. To cook the satay, thread the marinaded pork onto long wooden skewers or satay sticks. Line the grill rack with foil and grill for 5–6 minutes or until cooked, turning occasionally.

Total CHO Neg
Total Cals 1670

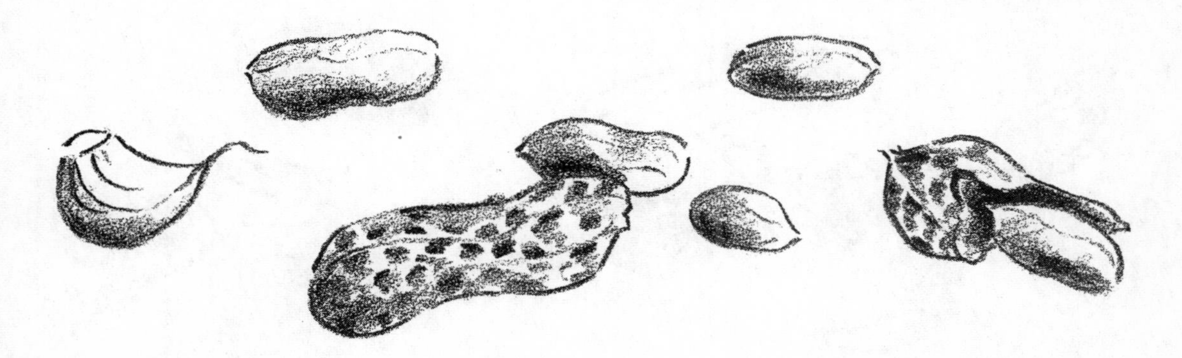

Chilli con Carne

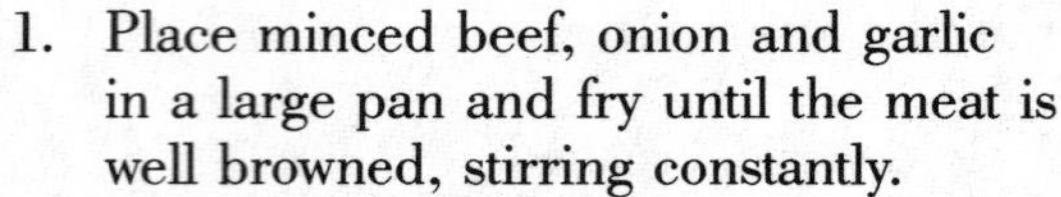

Serves 3–4

1 lb (455g) lean minced beef
1 onion, chopped
1 clove garlic, crushed
1–2 teaspoons (5–10ml) chilli powder
(to taste)
2 tablespoons (30ml) tomato purée
1×14 oz (400g) tin tomatoes
¼ pint (140ml) beef stock
Sea salt and freshly ground black pepper
1×15 oz (425g) tin red kidney beans,
drained and rinsed in cold water

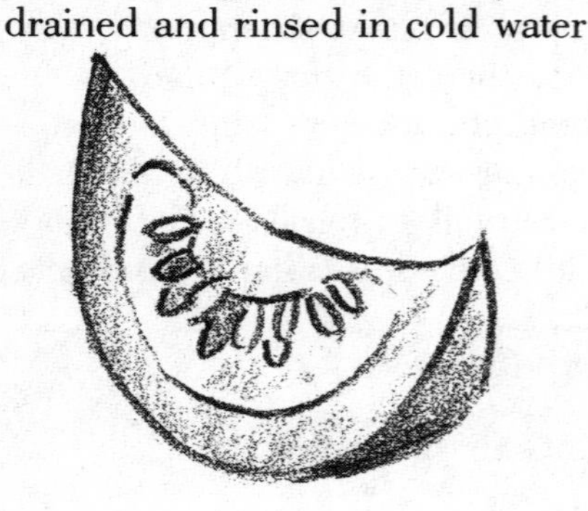

1. Place minced beef, onion and garlic in a large pan and fry until the meat is well browned, stirring constantly.
2. Stir in the chilli powder, tomato purée, tomatoes, stock and seasoning to taste and bring to the boil.
3. Reduce the heat, cover and simmer gently for 30 minutes, adding the kidney beans 10 minutes before the end of the cooking time. Adjust seasoning and serve.

NB: If you serve the Chilli with rice, don't forget to add on the extra carbohydrate and calories!

Total CHO 40g
Total Cals 1070

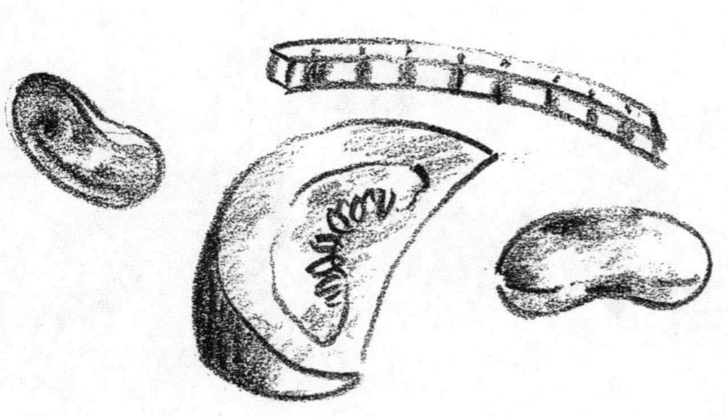

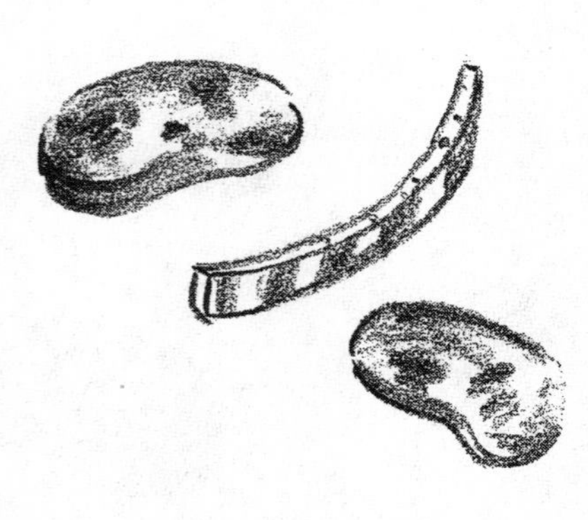

Pork in Cider and Mustard

Serves 4

2 tablespoons (30ml) corn or sunflower oil
4 boneless pork loin chops
2 onions, chopped
1 clove garlic, crushed
2 oz (55g) rindless streaky bacon
½ pint (285ml) dry cider
4 oz (115g) button mushrooms, sliced
3 tablespoons (45ml) coarse grain mustard
Sea salt and freshly ground black pepper
to taste
5 fl oz (142ml) carton soured cream

Total CHO Neg

Total Cals 1900

1. Heat the oil, add the chops and cook for approximately 2 minutes on each side. Remove and set aside.
2. Add the onion, garlic and bacon to the pan and sauté for 3 minutes. Add the cider and boil for 3 minutes or until reduced by a third.
3. Add the mushrooms and mustard and season to taste. Return the chops to the pan and spoon over the sauce. Reduce the heat and simmer for approximately 15 minutes or until the chops are tender.
4. Transfer the chops to a warmed serving dish. Keep warm. Stir the cream into the sauce and reheat gently — do not allow to boil.
5. Spoon the sauce over the chops and serve immediately.

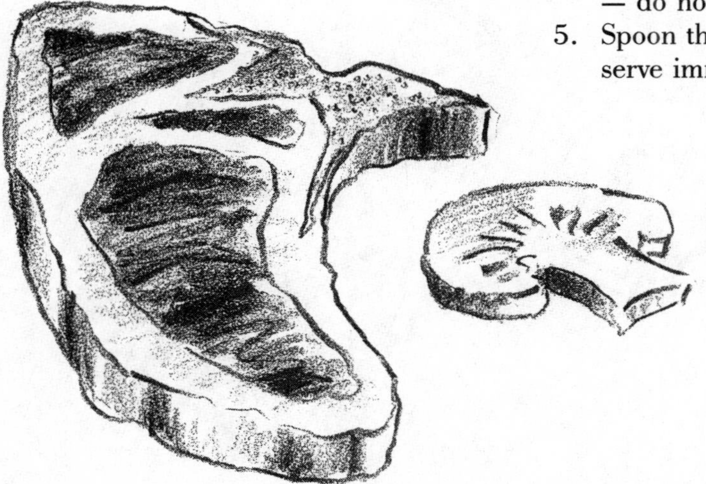

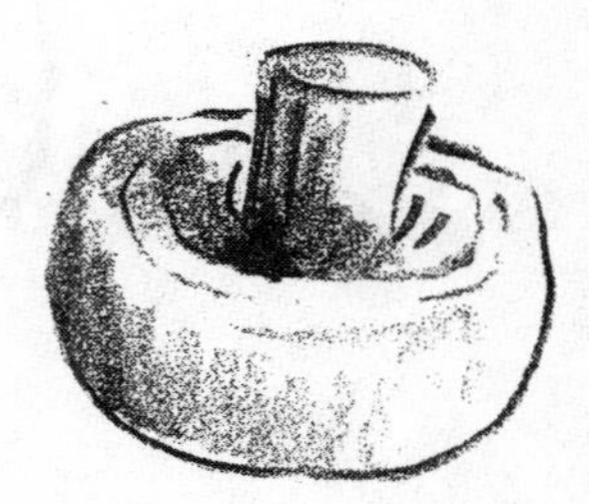

Beef Stroganoff

Serves 4

1–2 tablespoons (15–30ml) corn or sunflower oil
1 onion, finely chopped
8 oz (225g) button mushrooms, cleaned and sliced
1 lb (455g) fillet steak, cut into thin strips
1 teaspoon (5ml) Dijon mustard
Sea salt and freshly ground black pepper
2 tablespoons (30ml) brandy
5 fl oz (142ml) carton soured cream
Fresh parsley, chopped

Total CHO Neg

Total Cals 1270

1. Heat the oil, add the onion and fry for 5 minutes or until golden. Add the mushrooms and fry for a further 2 minutes.
2. Add the steak to the pan, stir in the mustard. Season well. Sauté briskly for 5 minutes or until the meat juices run pink.
3. Stir in the brandy and soured cream and heat through gently. Do not boil or the cream will curdle.
4. Adjust seasoning, transfer to a hot serving dish and sprinkle with parsley.

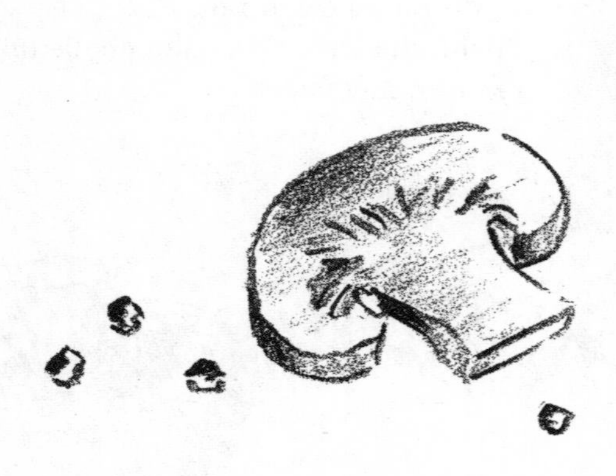

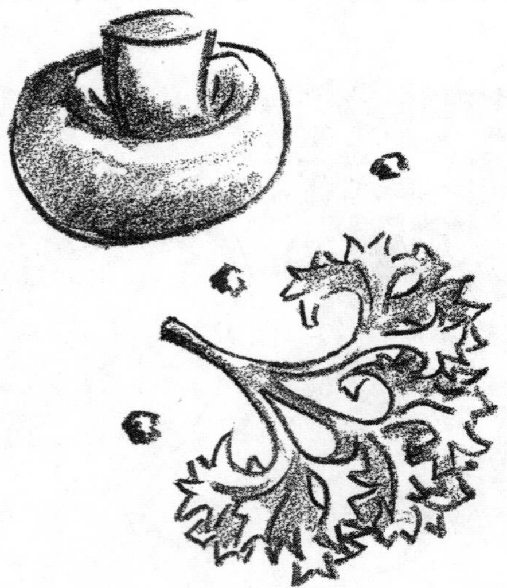

Boeuf Bourguignon

Serves 4

2 tablespoons (30ml) sunflower or corn oil
2 lb (905g) chuck steak
4 oz (115g) unsmoked bacon, rind removed and diced
1 tablespoon (15ml) wholemeal flour
Sea salt and freshly ground black pepper
½ pint (285ml) red wine
½ pint (285ml) beef stock
1 bouquet garni
8 oz (225g) small pickling onions
4 oz (115g) button mushrooms, sliced

Total CHO 10g
Total Cals 2080

1. Heat the oil in a flameproof casserole. Put in beef and brown quickly on all sides over high heat. Remove from the casserole and set aside.
2. Add the bacon to the casserole and fry for 2–3 minutes. Stir in the flour, add salt and pepper to taste and return the meat to the casserole.
3. Pour the wine and stock over the meat. Add the bouquet garni, cover the casserole and transfer to a warm oven 325°F/160°C (Gas Mark 3).
4. Cook for 2 hours. Add the onions and mushrooms approximately 40 minutes before the end of the cooking time.
5. Discard the bouquet garni and adjust the seasoning before serving.

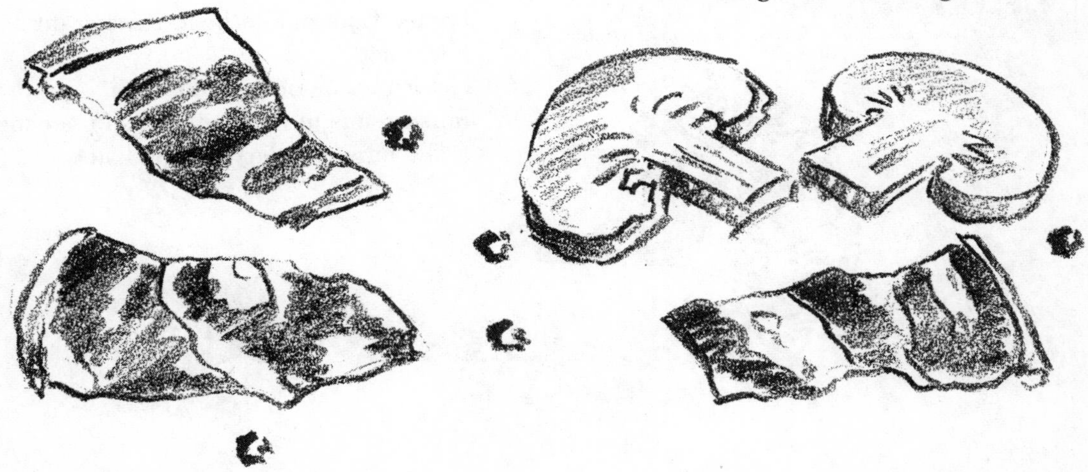

Escalopes of Pork à la Crème

Serves 4

4 thin escalopes of pork
2 tablespoons (30ml) corn or sunflower oil
1 onion, chopped
4 oz (115g) button mushrooms, thinly sliced
½ pint (285ml) chicken stock *or* ¼ pint (140ml) white wine and ¼ pint (140ml) chicken stock
4 fl oz (113ml) single cream
1 teaspoon (5ml) low-fat spread
1 teaspoon (5ml) flour
Sea salt and freshly ground black pepper
1 tablespoon (15ml) fresh parsley, chopped

Total CHO Neg

Total Cals 1560

1. Work together low-fat spread and flour to make beurre manié; set aside.
2. Flatten escalopes between 2 sheets of greaseproof paper using a rolling pin. Heat the oil and fry the escalopes 3–4 minutes each side. Remove from pan (keep warm).
3. Add onion and mushrooms and cook for 3–4 minutes. Remove from pan (keep warm).
4. Add half the stock. Reduce by half, swilling it well round. Add remaining stock and bring to the boil. Boil for one minute, strain, and return liquid to pan. Add cream. Boil for one minute. Remove from heat.
5. Add and stir in beurre manié in small knobs. Continue to heat, stirring until thickened.
6. Return escalopes, onions and mushrooms to the pan and simmer for a few minutes. Serve immediately.

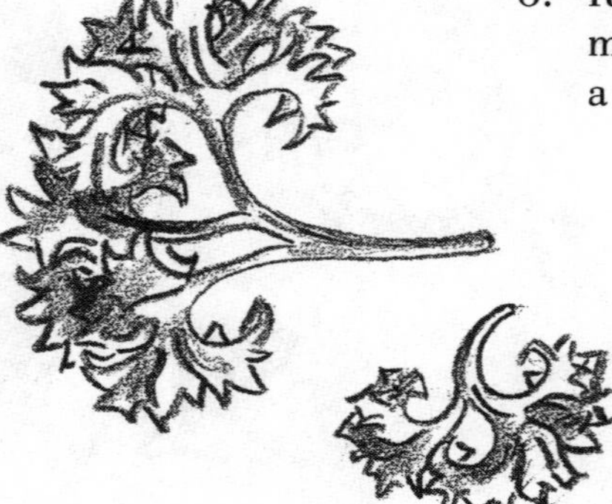

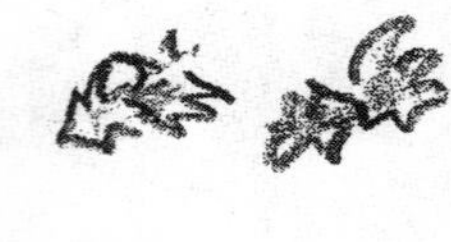

Spaghetti Bolognese

Serves 3–4

1 lb (455g) lean minced beef
1 onion, chopped
1 clove garlic, crushed
2 tablespoons (30ml) tomato purée
1×14 oz (400g) tin tomatoes
Approx. ½ pint (285ml) chicken stock
½ teaspoon (2.5ml) basil
½ teaspoon (2.5ml) oregano
Sea salt and freshly ground black pepper

Total CHO Neg

Total Cals 820

1. Add minced beef, onion and garlic to a large frying pan. Fry until browned, stirring constantly.
2. Stir in the tomato purée, tomatoes and stock and mix until well blended.
3. Stir in the remaining ingredients and season to taste. Bring to the boil.
4. Lower the heat and simmer gently for 20 minutes, stirring occasionally (adding a little more stock if the sauce becomes dry).
5. Serve immediately.

Spare Ribs

Serves 2–4

1 lb (455g) pork spare ribs
2 tablespoons (30ml) Hoi Sin sauce
2 tablespoons (30ml) dry sherry
1 tablespoon (15ml) soya sauce
1 tablespoon (15ml) intense sweetener
1 teaspoon (5ml) Chinese curry powder
3 spring onions

Total CHO Neg
Total Cals 1360

1. Place ribs in an ovenproof dish. Mix Hoi Sin sauce, sherry, soya sauce, sweetener and curry powder with 2 tablespoons (30ml) of water.
2. Brush the ribs with the sauce and leave to marinade for 2–4 hours in the refrigerator.
3. Roast in a hot oven at 450°F/230°C (Gas Mark 8) for 10 minutes, then reduce oven temperature to 350°F/180°C (Gas Mark 4) for 35–40 minutes.
4. Garnish with spring onion curls* and serve immediately.

* To make spring onion curls, see page 101.

Chicken Curry

Serves 4–6

2 tablespoons (30ml) corn or sunflower oil
4 chicken breasts, cut into pieces
1–2 onions, chopped
2 cloves garlic, crushed
2–3 tablespoons (30–45ml) curry powder
1 tablespoon (15ml) flour
2 tablespoons (30ml) tomato purée
Juice of ½ lemon
1 oz (30g) desiccated coconut
½ teaspoon (2.5ml) cinnamon
½ teaspoon (2.5ml) ground ginger
Pinch cayenne pepper
Bay leaf
2 tablespoons (30ml) mango chutney
Sea salt to taste
1 pint (570ml) water

1. Heat the oil and stir-fry the chicken over a high heat until lightly golden. Add the onion and garlic and cook for a further 5 minutes.
2. Stir in the curry powder, flour, tomato purée, lemon juice and coconut. Mix well.
3. Add remaining ingredients and bring to the boil, stirring continuously. Reduce heat and simmer gently for 30 minutes or until chicken is tender, and liquid has reduced, stirring frequently.
4. Serve hot.

Total CHO 20g

Total Cals 1320

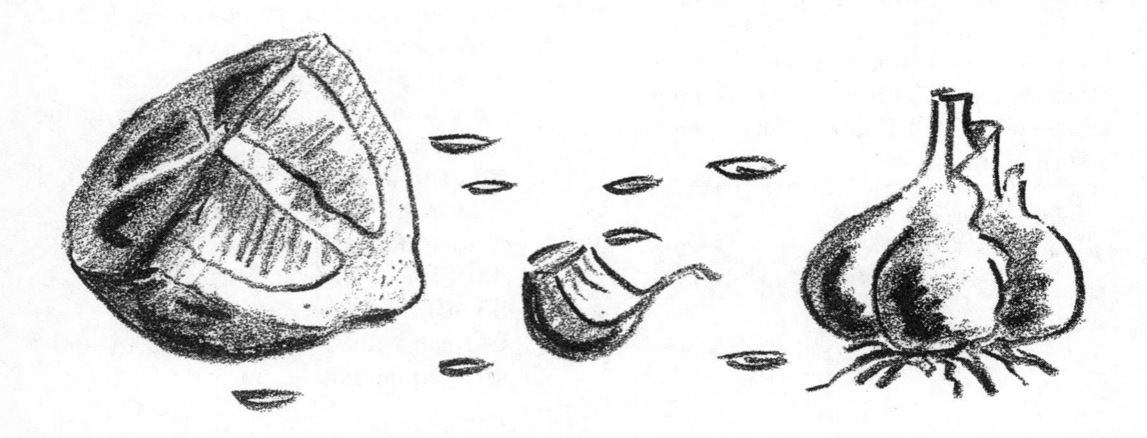

Turkey and Rice Ring

Serves 10

For the filling:

6 tablespoons (90ml) low-calorie mayonnaise
½ teaspoon (2.5ml) curry powder
1 oz (30g) unsalted cashew nuts
7 oz (200g) cooked turkey, chopped

For the rice:

9 oz (255g) brown rice, cooked
7 oz (200g) mixed vegetables, cooked — e.g. sweet corn, peppers, peas

For the dressing:

2 tablespoons (30ml) corn oil
1 tablespoon (15ml) wine vinegar
¼ teaspoon (1.25ml) dry mustard
Sprinkle of paprika to garnish

1. Combine the mayonnaise and curry powder. Mix well. Add the cashew nuts and turkey. Stir and season to taste.
2. Add the vegetables to the rice. Blend the corn oil, wine vinegar and mustard together and toss with the rice and vegetables.
3. Press into a lightly oiled 8-inch (20cm) ring mould. Turn out onto a flat serving plate and spoon the turkey mixture into the centre.
4. Sprinkle with a little paprika. Keep in refrigerator until served.

Total CHO 200g

Total Cals 940

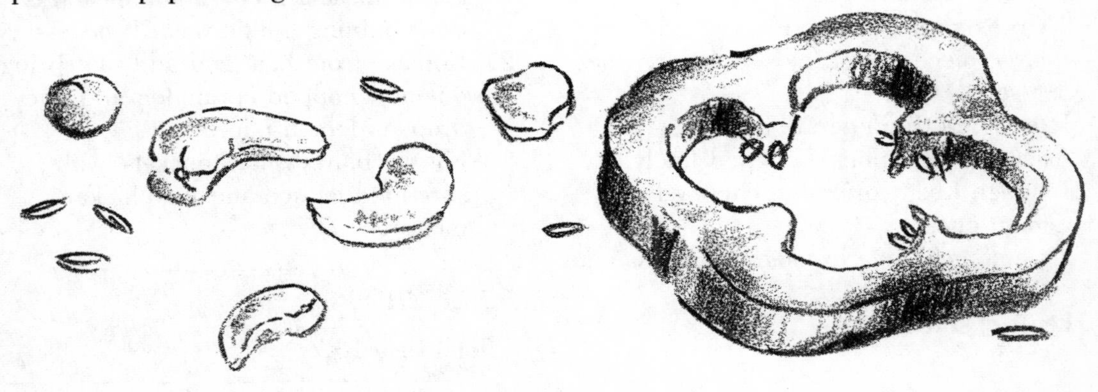

Stir-fried Turkey

Serves 4

2 tablespoons (30ml) oil
1–2 teaspoons (5–10ml) cumin seeds
1 bunch spring onions or 1 large onion, chopped
1 clove garlic, crushed
3 small peppers, red, yellow and green, chopped
4 oz (115g) broccoli heads
4 oz (115g) mushrooms, sliced
9 oz (255g) cooked turkey, chopped

1. Heat the oil in a large pan or wok and add the cumin seeds. Fry for a few seconds.
2. Add the onion and garlic. Stir. Add the peppers and broccoli and cook for 1–2 minutes. Add the mushrooms and turkey and toss to combine all the ingredients and cook until the turkey is hot.
3. Serve immediately.

Total CHO Neg

Total Cals 630

Chicken Pockets

Serves 4

1 tablespoon (15ml) polyunsaturated oil
1 lb (455g) chicken, minced
2–3 green chillies, chopped
3 cloves garlic, crushed
1 large piece ginger, peeled and crushed
Sea salt to taste
1 teaspoon (5ml) garam masala
A few spring onions, chopped finely
1 bunch fresh coriander, chopped
Lemon juice
2 wholemeal pitta breads, cut across into 2 halves or 'pockets'
Lettuce, shredded

1. Heat the oil and add the chicken with the chillies, garlic, ginger, salt, and garam masala. Cook until chicken is done, adding a little water if necessary.
2. Remove from heat and add the spring onions, chopped coriander, and a few drops of lemon juice.
3. Fill the halved pitta 'pockets' with shredded lettuce and the chicken mixture.

Total CHO 80g

Total Cals 1020

Chicken and Celery

Serves 2–4

8 oz (225g) chicken breast, sliced
Pinch of salt
1 tablespoon (15ml) cornflour
2–3 tablespoons (30–45ml) corn or sunflower oil
4 slices root ginger, chopped
3 spring onions, chopped
1 stick celery, chopped
1 small green pepper, cut into small strips
2 tablespoons (30ml) soya sauce
1 tablespoon (15ml) dry sherry

Total CHO 10g
Total Cals 700

1. Mix the chicken with the salt and cornflour. Heat the oil in a wok and stir-fry the chicken over moderate heat until the pieces are lightly coloured. Remove the chicken.
2. Increase the heat and add the root ginger, spring onions, celery, and green pepper. Stir continuously for about 30 seconds, then add the chicken with the soya sauce and sherry.
3. Cook for a further 1–1½ minutes, stirring well.
4. Serve hot.

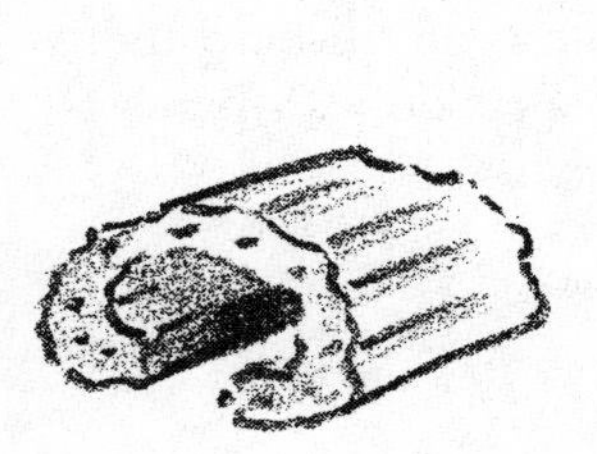

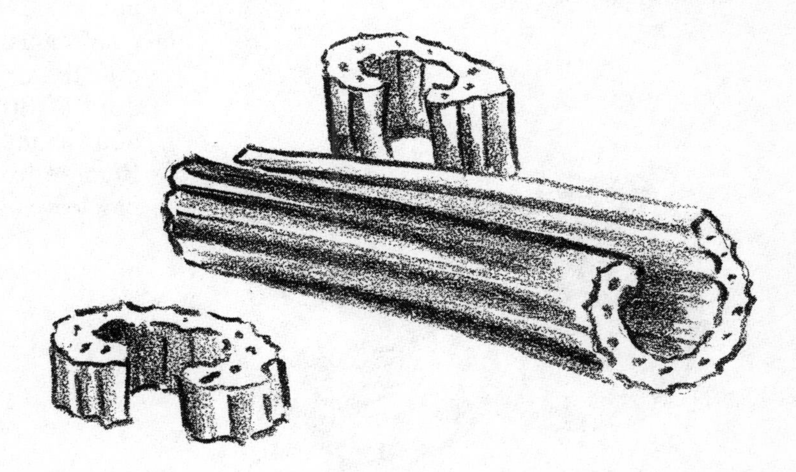

Coq au Vin

Serves 4

2 tablespoons (30ml) sunflower oil
4 oz (115g) streaky bacon
2 medium onions, chopped
1 clove garlic, crushed
6 oz (170g) button mushrooms
4 chicken breasts, skinned
2 tablespoons (30ml) dry sherry
2 level teaspoons (10ml) wholemeal flour
½ pint (285ml) red wine
¼ pint (140ml) chicken stock
2 bay leaves
Sea salt and freshly ground black pepper
Freshly chopped parsley

Total CHO 20g

Total Cals 1550

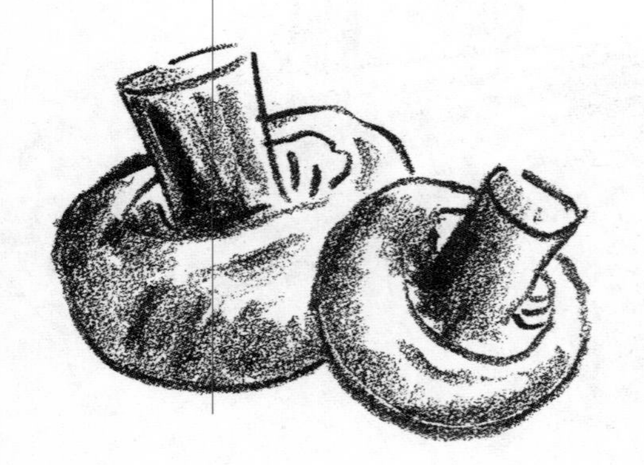

1. Heat 1 tablespoon (15ml) of oil in a large frying pan and stir-fry the bacon, onions, garlic, and mushrooms for 2–3 minutes. Remove from pan and put to one side.
2. Fry the chicken in remaining oil for 10 minutes until sealed and golden brown on both sides. Pour the sherry over the chicken and cook for approximately 1 minute.
3. Remove chicken and place in a casserole dish with bacon, mushrooms, onions and bay leaves.
4. Stir the flour carefully into the sherry to make a smooth sauce and cook for 2 minutes. Gradually stir in the wine and stock. Bring to the boil, stirring continuously and season to taste. Pour over the chicken, cover and cook at 350°F/180°C (Gas Mark 4) for 1 hour or until the chicken is tender.
5. Remove from the oven, discard the bay leaves and sprinkle with parsley.

Chicken à la King

Serves 4

1 oz (30g) low-fat spread
1 oz (30g) wholemeal flour
½ pint (285ml) skimmed milk
Sea salt and freshly ground black pepper
1 tablespoon (15ml) corn oil
1 small red or green pepper, finely chopped
1 onion, chopped
8 oz (225g) chicken breast, cooked

1. Make the sauce by melting the margarine, stir in the flour and blend in the milk. Stir continually until the sauce thickens and season to taste.
2. Heat the oil and lightly sauté the pepper, onion and chicken for 5–10 minutes.
3. Stir into the sauce and mix well.
4. Serve immediately.

Total CHO 35g
Total Cals 750

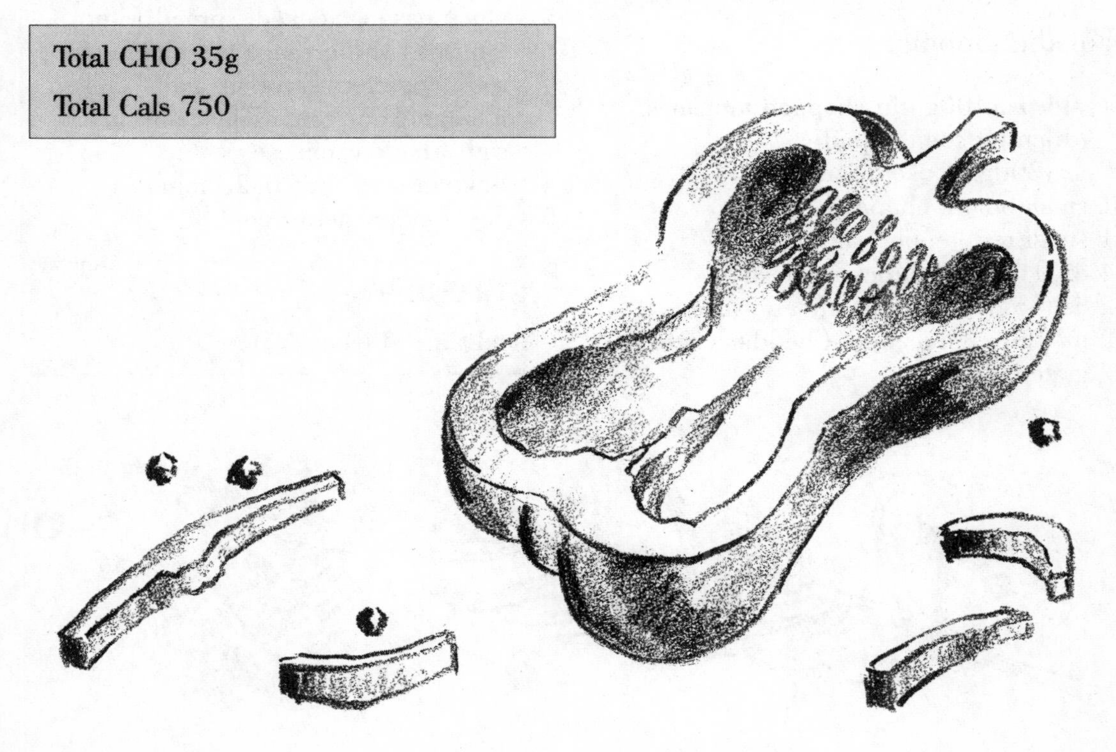

Ham and Mozzarella Pizza

Serves 6

For the base:

4 oz (115g) wholemeal self-raising flour
1 teaspoon (5ml) baking powder
1 oz (30g) low-fat spread
½ teaspoon (2.5ml) mixed herbs
1 small onion, finely chopped
1 egg
Skimmed milk to bind

For the topping:

1×14 oz (400g) tin chopped tomatoes, (drain off some liquid)
7 oz (200g) cooked ham
1 small onion, chopped
1 small red pepper, sliced
4 oz (115g) mushrooms, sliced
2 oz (55g) mozzarella cheese, sliced
2 oz (55g) reduced-fat Cheddar cheese, grated

1. Sieve the flour and baking powder. Rub in fat until the mixture resembles fine breadcrumbs. Add onion and herbs. Bind with egg and milk to form a dough.
2. Roll out to line a 9-inch (23cm) circle and bake in preheated oven, at 400°F/200°C (Gas Mark 6) for about 10 minutes.
3. Once base is cooked, spread with tomatoes and arrange the ham, onion, red pepper, mushrooms and mozzarella on top. Finally, sprinkle with Cheddar cheese.
4. Bake in oven for 20–25 minutes.
5. Serve either hot or cold.

Total CHO 90g
Total Cals 1140

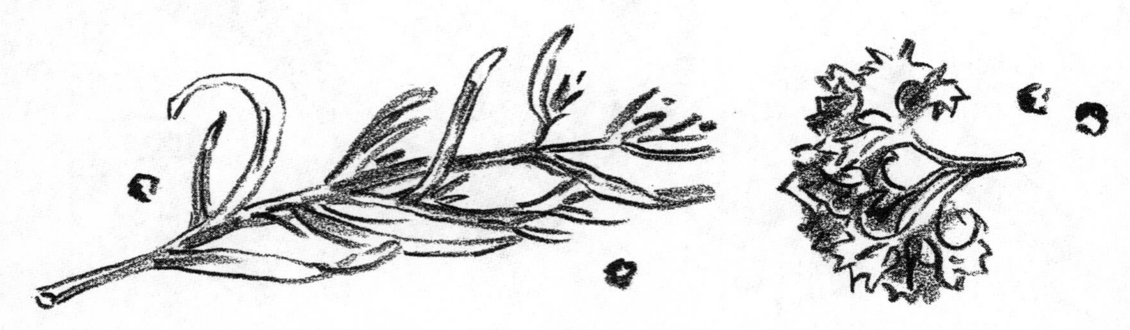

Asparagus Quiche

Serves 8

For the pastry:

4 oz (115g) wholemeal flour
2 oz (55g) plain flour
2 oz (55g) low-fat spread
1 oz (30g) vegetable fat
3 tablespoons (45ml) water

For the filling:

4 oz (115g) lean cooked ham, chopped
3 size 3 eggs
¼ pint (140ml) skimmed milk
1 oz (30g) reduced-fat Cheddar cheese, grated
Sea salt and freshly ground black pepper
1 small tin asparagus tips, drained

1. Make pastry and line a 9-inch (23cm) flan ring. Bake blind at 400°F/200°C (Gas Mark 6) for 10 minutes.
2. Cover the base of the flan ring with the chopped ham.
3. In a bowl, combine the eggs, milk, grated cheese and seasonings, and beat well to blend. Pour the mixture over the ham. Arrange the asparagus tips, pointed ends towards the centre, around the edge of the filling.
4. Bake the quiche in the centre of a 400°F/200°C (Gas Mark 6) oven for 35–40 minutes or until the filling is set and firm, and golden brown on top.

Total CHO 130g

Total Cals 1560

GOING VEGETARIAN

Vegetables supply a significant amount of fibre and vitamin C. Try to leave the skins on vegetables and to keep them whole rather than puréeing them. If left intact, the fibre can more effectively minimize fluctuations in blood sugar levels — something that is particularly important for people with diabetes. Vitamin C is easily destroyed by heat and light. To preserve it, boil in the minimum amount of water or steam vegetables for the shortest possible time in a pan with a tight-fitting lid, and serve immediately. Eating vegetables raw is even better.

Many people are unaccustomed to eating pulses such as beans and lentils. These recipes will introduce you to the wide range of different colours and shapes of pulses which can be used to increase the protein and fibre content of savoury dishes. Their protein content is particularly important for vegetarians and vegans. On soaking, pulses almost double in size and so can be very economical — taste without waste!

Green Beans and Tomato

Serves 4

1 tablespoon (15ml) corn or sunflower oil
1 onion, chopped
1 lb (455g) tomatoes, skinned and chopped
1 lb (455g) green beans, cooked
Sea salt and freshly ground black pepper to taste
Small bunch fresh coriander, chopped

1. Heat the oil and sauté the onion for 5 minutes.
2. Stir in the tomatoes and beans.
3. Season to taste. Sprinkle with chopped coriander. Serve hot.

Total CHO Neg

Total Cals 230

Julienne Carrots

Serves 4–6

1 lb (455g) carrots, peeled and cut into julienne strips
1 onion, grated
½-inch (1cm) piece fresh root ginger, grated
Sea salt and freshly ground black pepper to taste
1 tablespoon (15ml) lemon juice
1 tablespoon (15ml) fresh parsley, chopped

1. Place all ingredients except parsley in a pan and add enough water just to cover them.
2. Simmer for 10–15 minutes, until all the liquid has evaporated.
3. Serve immediately, sprinkled with chopped parsley.

Total CHO Neg

Total Cals 100

Creamed Sprouts

Serves 6

2 lb (905g) Brussels sprouts, cooked until tender (conserve liquid)
4 oz (115g) low-fat soft cheese
Sea salt and freshly ground black pepper to taste
Grated nutmeg to taste
1 tablespoon (15ml) flaked almonds

Total CHO Neg

Total Cals 480

1. Purée the sprouts and cheese in a food processor or electric blender until smooth. Add a little of the vegetable cooking liquid if the purée is too dry.
2. Season to taste. Transfer to a warmed serving dish.
3. Sprinkle with the almonds. Grill until almonds are toasted. Serve immediately.

Potatoes Layered

Serves 6

2 lb (905g) potatoes, peeled and thinly sliced
1 large onion, sliced
Sea salt and freshly ground black pepper to taste
Grated nutmeg to taste
1 pint (570ml) chicken stock
1 oz (30g) low-fat spread, melted
1-2 oz (30-55g) half-fat hard cheese

Total CHO 160g
Total Cals 860

1. In a shallow dish, layer the potato and onion, seasoning well and finishing with a layer of potato slices.
2. Pour in the stock and brush the potatoes with the low-fat spread.
3. Sprinkle with the cheese and cook at 350°F/180°C (Gas Mark 4) for approximately 1½ hours, until cooked and crisp on top.
4. Serve immediately.

Braised Cabbage

Serves 4

1 tablespoon (15ml) corn or sunflower oil
1 onion, chopped
1 clove garlic, crushed
1 lb (455g) red cabbage, shredded
1 medium cooking apple, peeled and sliced
3 tablespoons (45ml) wine vinegar
3 tablespoons (45ml) water
Sea salt and freshly ground black pepper

Total CHO Neg
Total Cals 200

1. Heat the oil and sauté the onion and garlic.
2. Add the cabbage and apple and cook for 5 minutes.
3. Spoon into an ovenproof dish. Add the vinegar and water. Cover with foil. Cook at 350°F/180°C (Gas Mark 4) for about 45 minutes.
4. Drain and serve immediately.

Rumble de Thumps

Serves 4–6

1 lb (455g) potatoes, cooked and creamed with ½ oz (15g) low-fat spread and 1 tablespoon (15ml) skimmed milk
1 lb (455g) green cabbage, cooked
1 onion, finely chopped
Sea salt and freshly ground black pepper
1 oz (30g) vegetarian Cheddar cheese, grated

1. Mix the potato, cabbage and onion. Season and place in an ovenproof dish.
2. Sprinkle on the grated cheese. Bake at 375°F/190°C (Gas Mark 5) for 30–40 minutes.

Total CHO 80g

Total Cals 510

Stuffed Peppers

Serves 4

4 medium size peppers (assorted colours)
3 oz (85g) brown rice, cooked
4oz (115g) mixed vegetables
4 oz (115g) frozen sweet corn
1 onion, finely chopped
1 teaspoon (5ml) mixed herbs
Sea salt and freshly ground black pepper

Total CHO 80g

Total Cals 300

1. Slice the tops off peppers and retain the tops. Remove the cores and deseed the peppers, and place them in boiling water for 3–5 minutes.
2. Meanwhile, mix the remaining ingredients together. Season to taste.
3. Divide the mixture between the peppers, replace tops and place them in an ovenproof dish. Bake at 400°F/200°C (Gas Mark 6) for 25–30 minutes.

Makkai (Spicy Sweet Corn)

Serves 4

3 corn on the cob, cut into 2-inch (5cm) pieces
1 tablespoon (15ml) corn oil
2 teaspoons (10ml) cumin seeds
2 medium onions, chopped
4–6 cloves garlic, crushed
1 green chilli, chopped
½ teaspoon (2.5ml) garam masala
1 teaspoon (5ml) turmeric
1×8 oz (225g) tin tomatoes
1 tablespoon (15ml) lemon juice
Freshly chopped coriander leaves

1. Boil the sweet corn until cooked.
2. Heat the oil and fry the cumin seeds until they crackle.
3. Add the onion, garlic, and chilli and fry for 2–3 minutes. Stir in the garam masala, turmeric and tomatoes, and cook for about 5 minutes before adding the lemon juice.
4. Just before serving, add some fresh chopped coriander.

Total CHO 60g

Total Cals 280

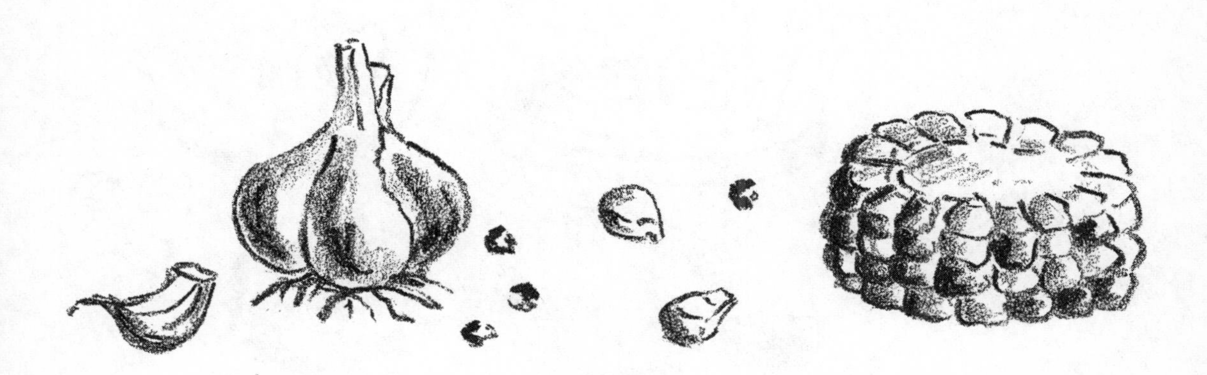

Mung Dhal

Serves 3–4

5 oz (140g) mung dhal (soaked in water overnight), drained
1 tablespoon (15ml) polyunsaturated oil
1 onion, chopped
1 clove garlic, crushed
1 teaspoon (5ml) ground coriander
1 teaspoon (5ml) ground cumin
1–2 green chillies, seeded and chopped
½ teaspoon (2.5ml) turmeric
Sea salt
1×8 oz (225g) tin tomatoes
Chopped coriander leaves

Total CHO 50g
Total Cals 470

1. Cover the dhal with water, bring to the boil then simmer until tender — about 20 minutes. (To give a little flavour try adding an onion impregnated with cloves to the cooking liquid.)
2. Heat the oil and fry the onion and garlic until tender. Add the coriander, cumin, chillies, turmeric, salt and tomatoes. Stir and cook for about 10 minutes.
3. Stir in the lightly drained dhal and cook for a further 10 minutes on a low heat.
4. When ready add the chopped coriander leaves.

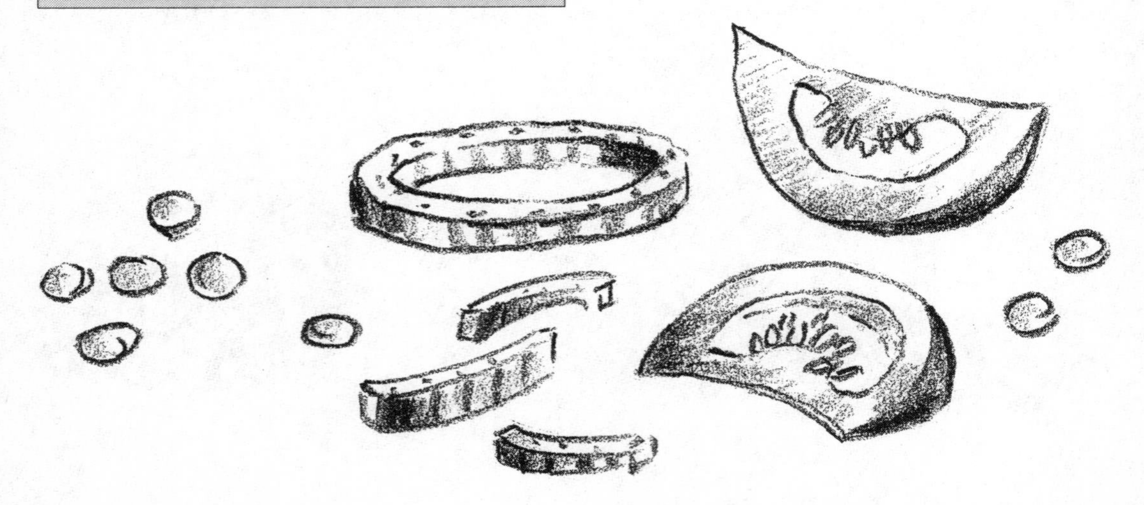

Courgette and Tomato Pie

Serves 4

2 tablespoons (30ml) corn or sunflower oil
1 lb (455g) courgettes, sliced
2 onions, sliced
2 cloves garlic, crushed
1×14 oz (400g) tin tomatoes
1 tablespoon (15ml) tomato purée
Sea salt and freshly ground black pepper

For the topping:

1 lb (455g) potatoes, boiled and mashed
2 oz (55g) vegetarian Cheddar cheese, grated

1. Heat the oil and fry the courgettes, onions, and garlic for approximately 10 minutes, stirring occasionally.
2. Add the tomatoes and tomato purée. Season to taste. Cook for a further 5 minutes. Transfer to an ovenproof dish.
3. Spoon the mashed potato over the courgette mixture. Sprinkle with grated cheese. Bake at 400°F/200°C (Gas Mark 6) for 30–40 minutes.

Total CHO 80g

Total Cals 840

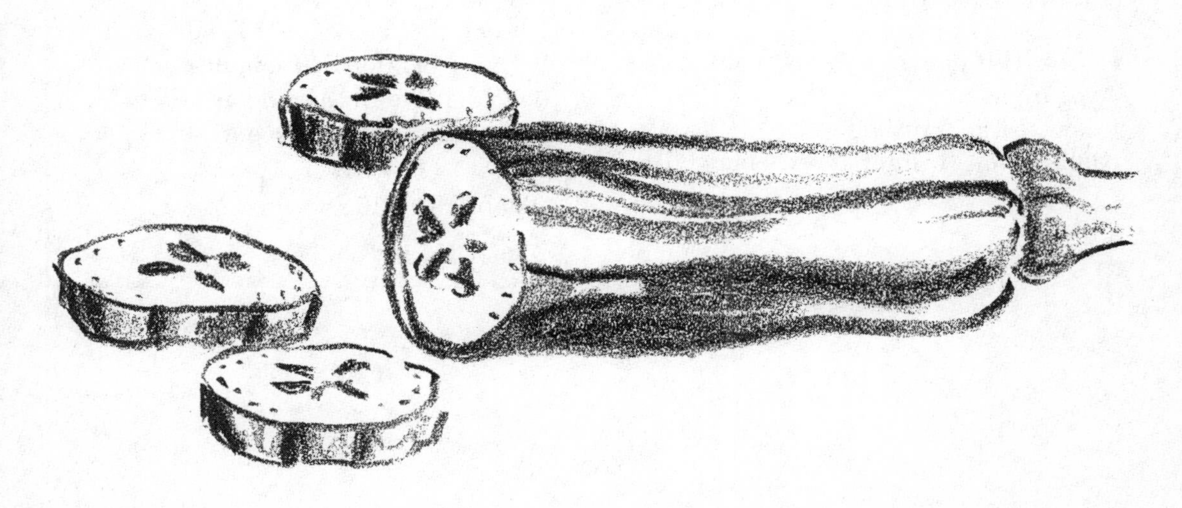

Lentil Rissoles with Yogurt Dressing

Makes 8–12

1 tablespoon (15ml) corn or sunflower oil
1 onion, finely chopped
2 carrots, finely chopped
2 sticks celery, finely chopped
8 oz (225g) Continental lentils, washed
1 pint (570ml) water
Sea salt and freshly ground black pepper
2 tablespoons (30ml) fresh parsley, chopped
1 teaspoon (5ml) ground coriander
1 teaspoon (5ml) ground cumin
1 tablespoon (15ml) tomato purée
6 oz (170g) wholemeal breadcrumbs
1 oz (30g) wholemeal flour
1 size 3 egg, beaten

For the dressing:

1×5 oz (140g) carton low-fat natural yogurt
1 clove garlic, crushed
1 tablespoon (15ml) parsley, chopped

1. Heat the oil and fry the onion, carrots and celery for 5 minutes. Add the lentils and water. Bring to the boil and simmer for approximately 50 minutes, stirring occasionally. (The lentils should be soft and no water visible).
2. Season to taste. Add the parsley, spices, tomato purée and 2 oz (55g) of the breadcrumbs. Allow to cool.
3. To shape the rissoles, divide the mixture into 8 or 12. Shape into patties (beefburger shape).
4. Roll each patty in the flour, dip in the egg and roll in the breadcrumbs. Repeat until all rissoles are formed. Chill in refrigerator for approximately 1 hour.
4. Cook the rissoles in a lightly oiled frying pan for 5–8 minutes until golden brown, turning occasionally.
5. Serve hot with the yogurt dressing.

Total CHO 220g

Total Cals 1440

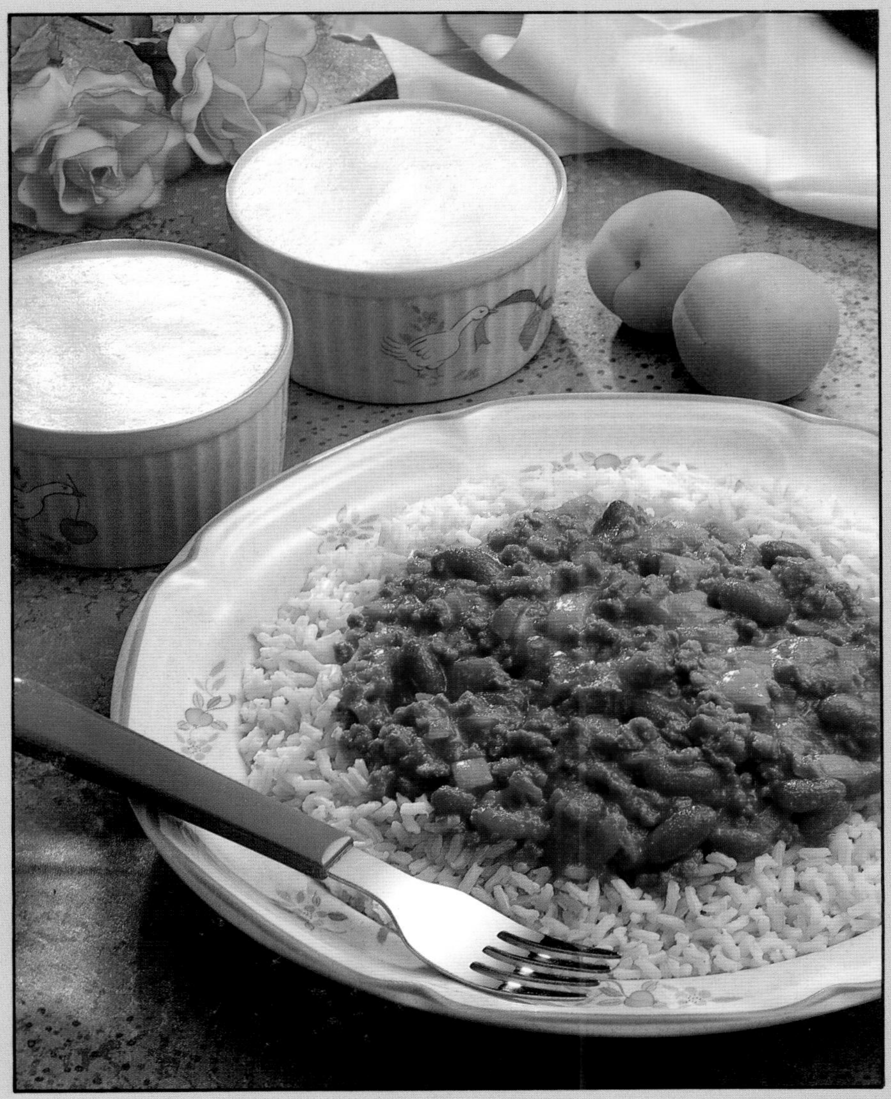

Chilli con Carne (page 42), served here with brown rice, makes a filling main meal for a winter's day. And if you have any room left, try Apricot Creams (page 87).

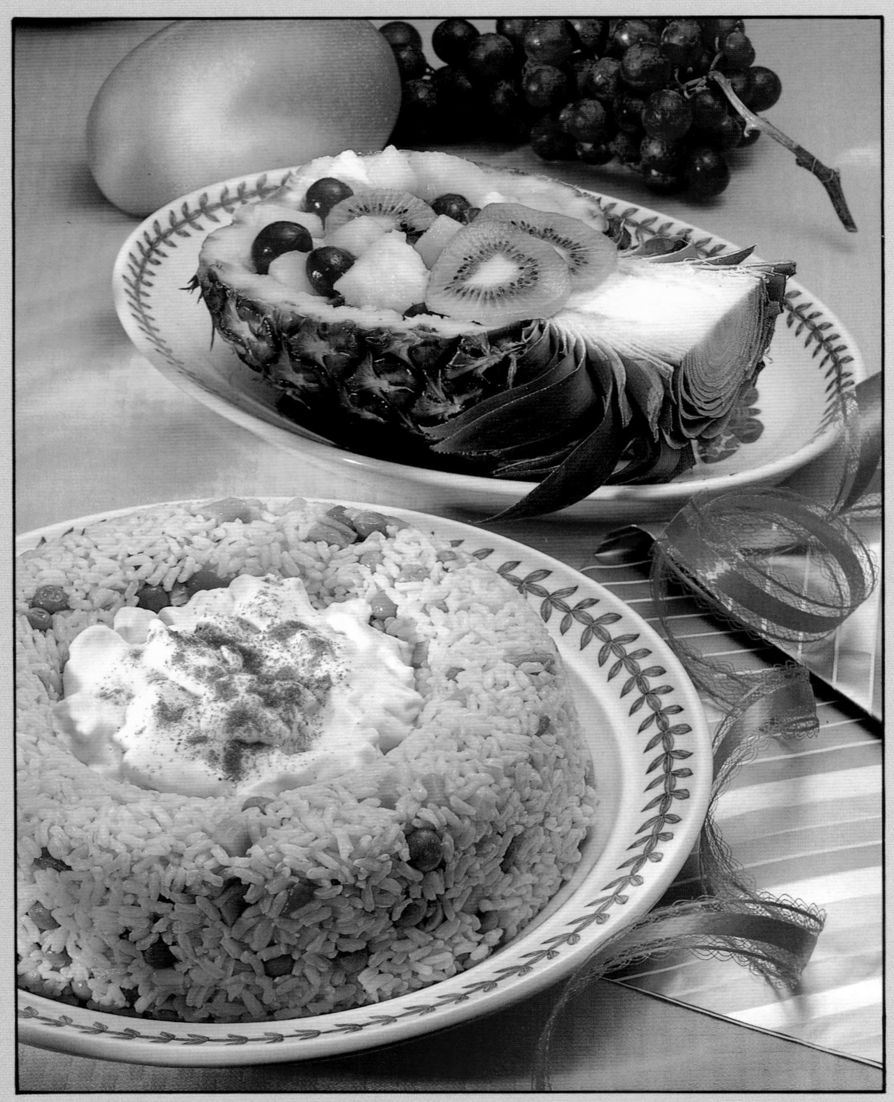

Perfect for a special celebration: Turkey and Rice Ring (page 49) and Tropical Pineapple Boats (page 93).

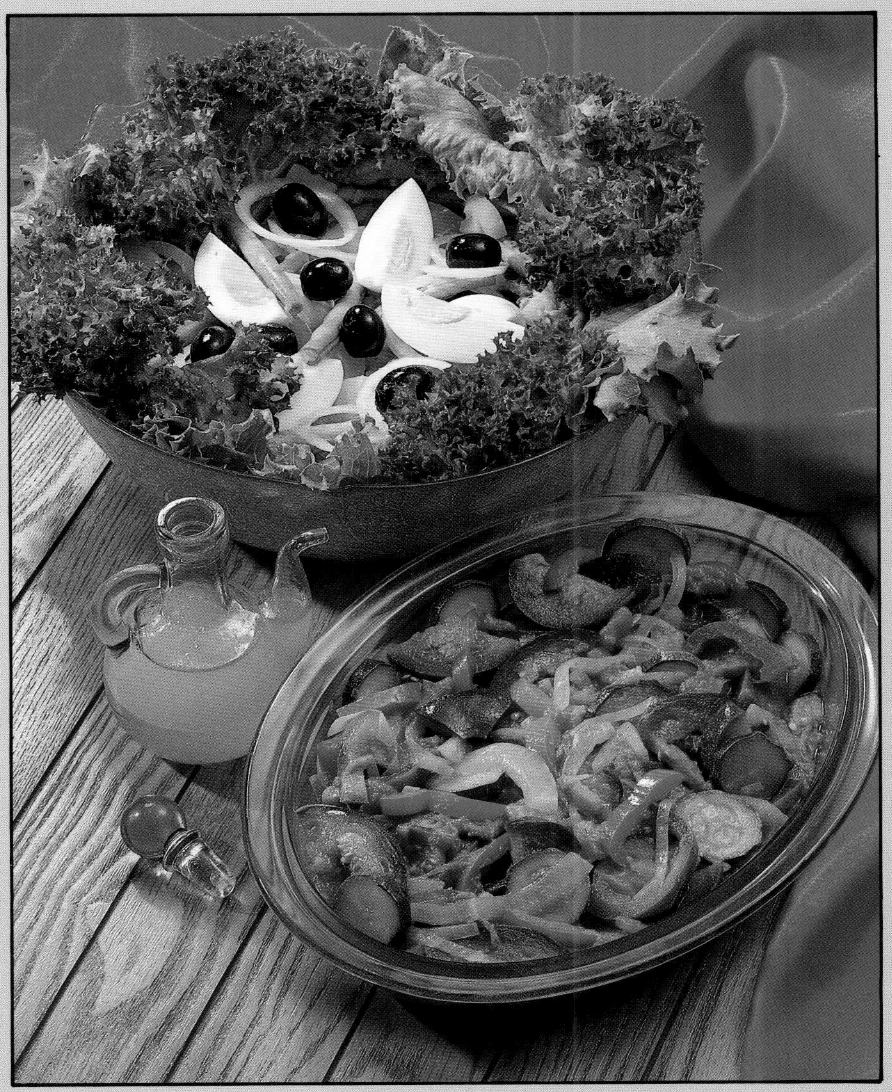

A low-calorie lunch with a Mediterranean feel: Ratatouille (page 76) and Salade Niçoise (page 79).

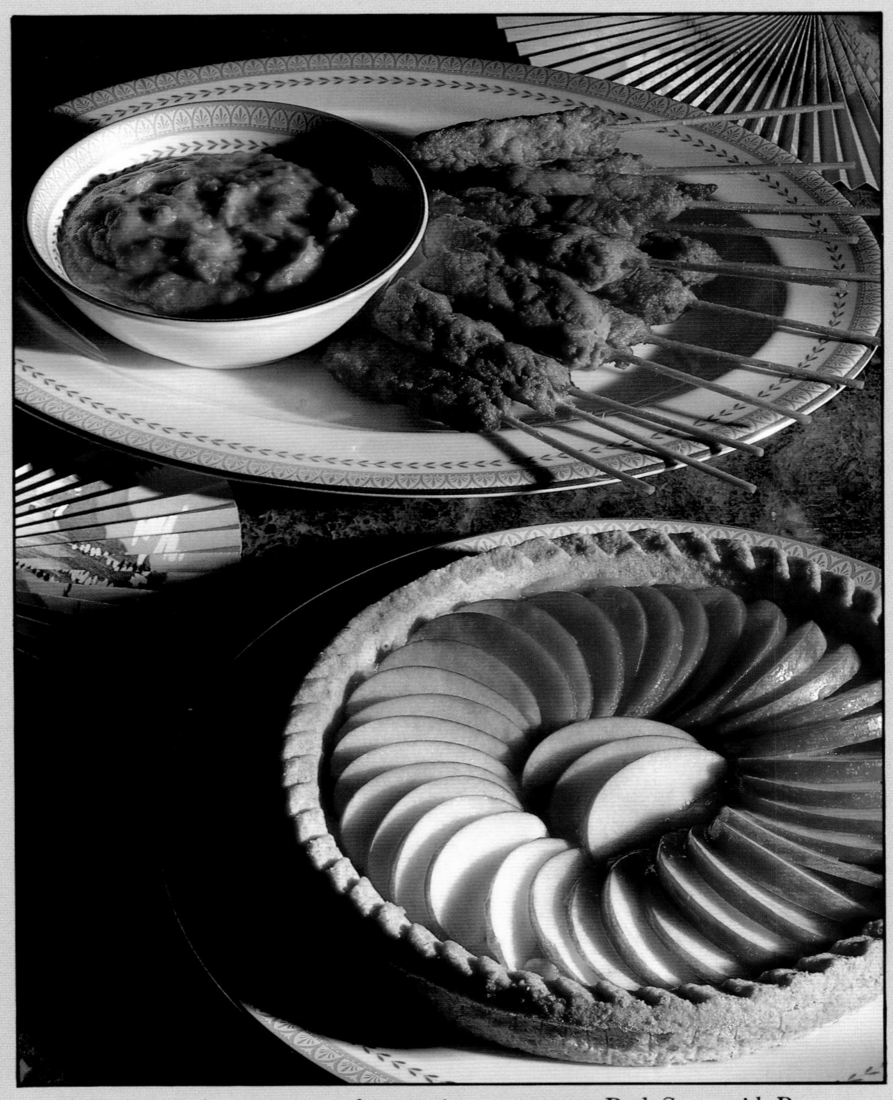

For a special dinner party, why not give your guests Pork Satay with Peanut Sauce (page 41) followed by French Apple Flan (page 94)?

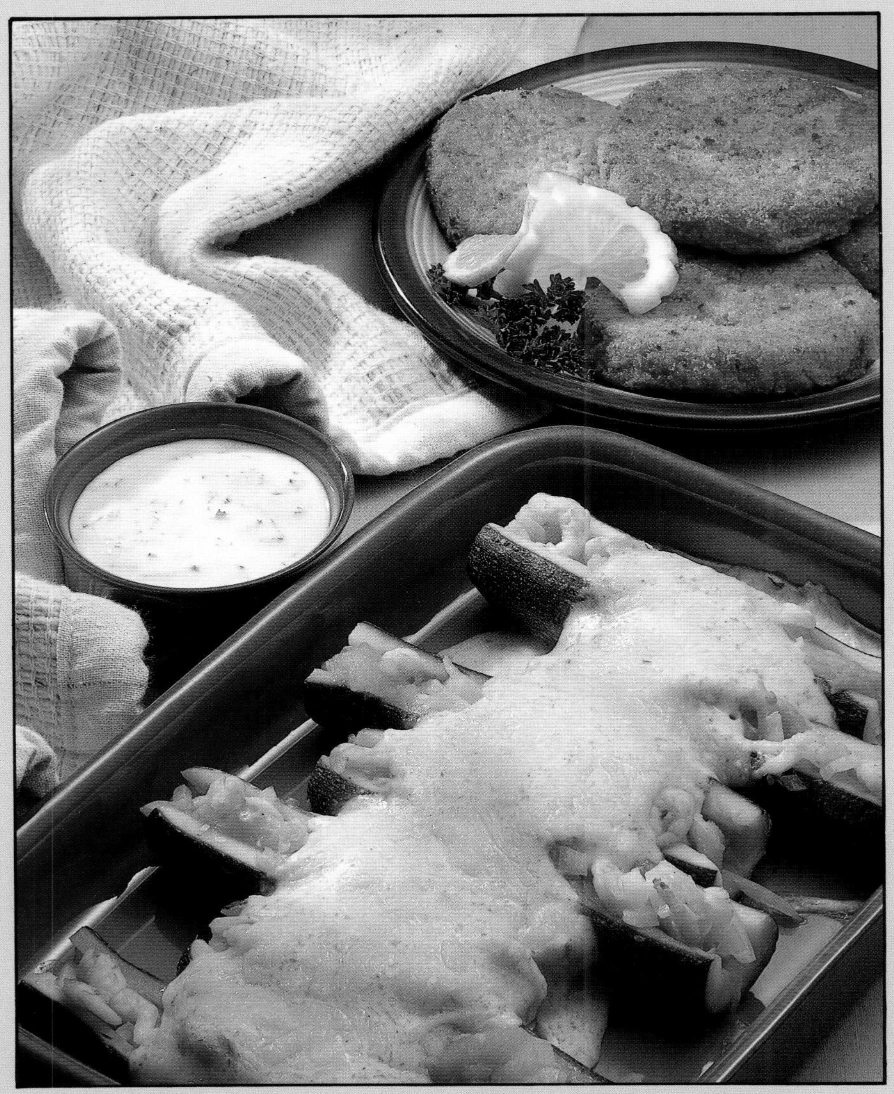

If you're in the process of going vegetarian, or if you don't eat red meat, try Courgettes Maison (page 28) and Lentil Rissoles with Yogurt Dressing (page 64).

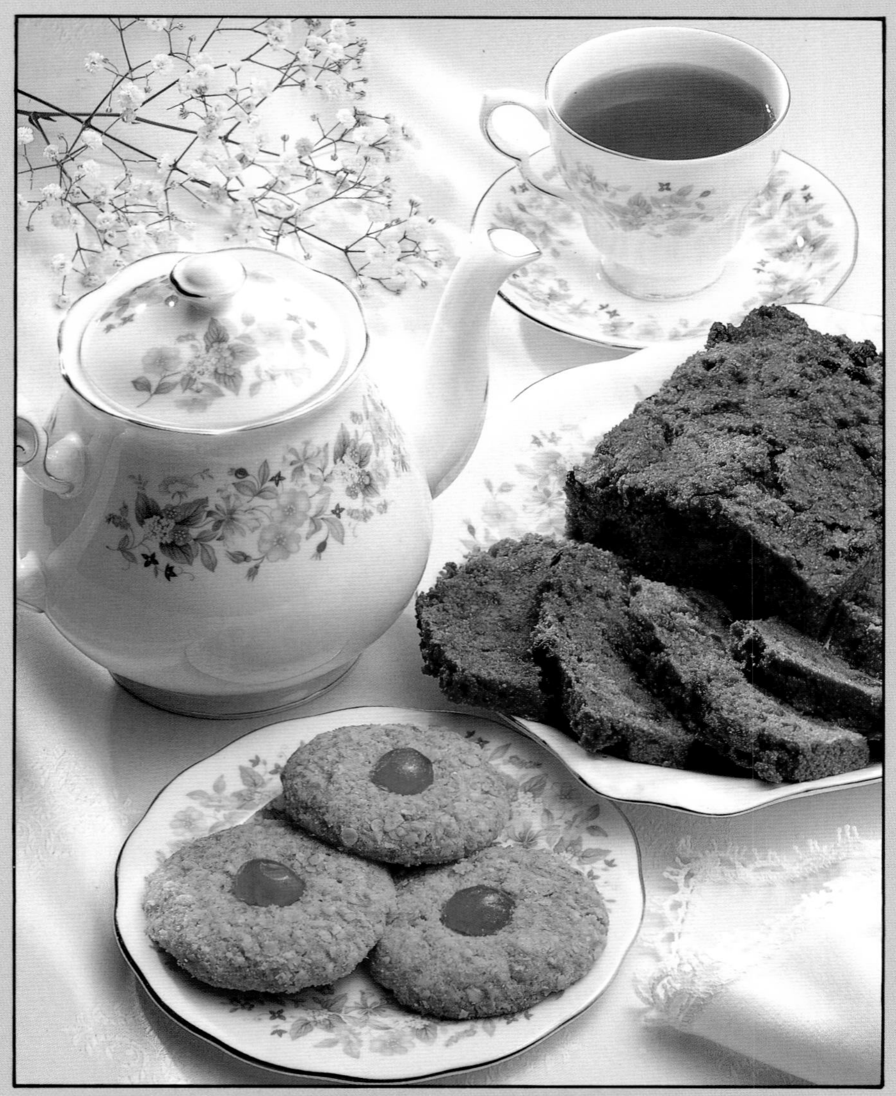

Next time friends pop round for afternoon tea, offer them home-baked Bran Fruit Loaf (page 97) and Melting Moments (page 100).

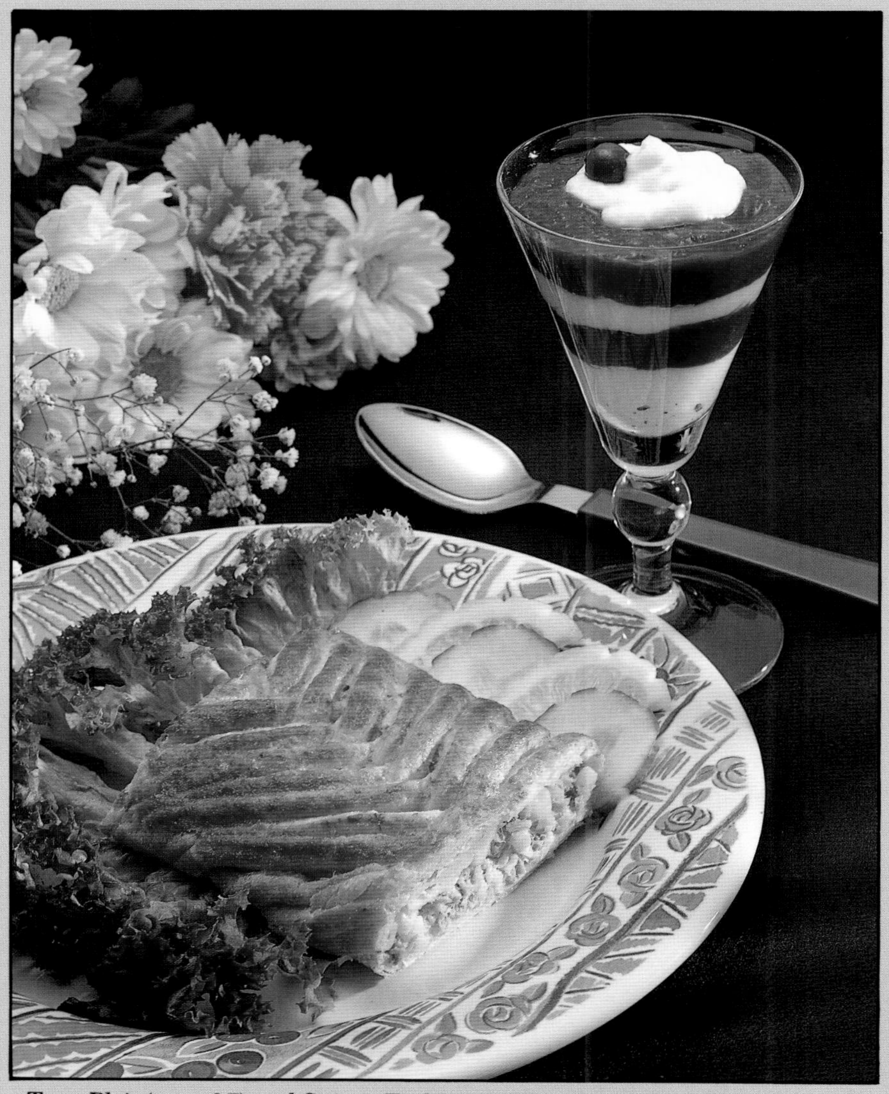

Tuna Plait (page 37) and Stripey Fool (page 85) make an ideal late supper for your guests.

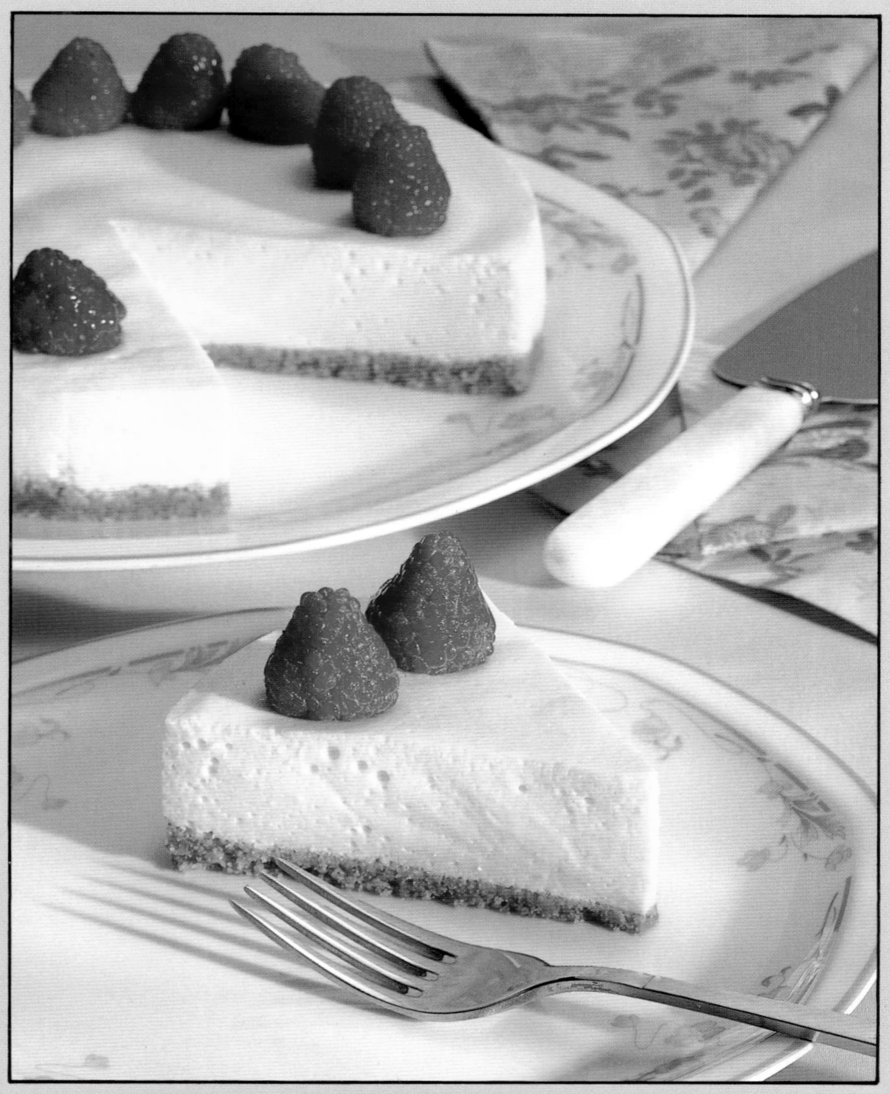

Cheesecake is a perennial favourite, and you can eat this one (page 91) with a perfectly clear conscience!

Spinach and Lentil Roulade

Serves 4–6

3 oz (85g) lentils
1 small onion, chopped
1 tablespoon (15ml) tomato purée
½ teaspoon (2.5ml) cumin (optional)
Sea salt and freshly ground black pepper
1 lb (455g) frozen spinach, defrosted
1 oz (30g) low-fat margarine
1 oz (30g) wholemeal flour
½ pint (285ml) skimmed milk
2 size 3 eggs, separated

Total CHO 70g

Total Cals 935

1. Grease and line an 11-inch (28cm) Swiss roll tin. Cook the lentils and onion until tender. Drain well. Return to the pan and heat to evaporate any excess moisture.
2. Add the tomato purée and cumin, if using. Sieve or purée. Adjust the seasoning and set aside.
3. Cook the spinach without water for 3–4 minutes. Turn it into a colander or sieve and press well to remove as much liquid as possible.
4. To make the white sauce, melt the margarine, stir in the flour. Add the milk and bring to the boil stirring until the sauce thickens. Stir in the spinach and egg yolks. Season.
5. Whisk egg whites until stiff and gently fold them into the spinach mixture. Spoon into the prepared tin. Level. Bake at 400°F/200°C (Gas Mark 6) for 20 minutes or until golden brown.
6. Turn out onto a sheet of greaseproof paper. Spread the lentil purée over the surface and roll up like a Swiss roll.
7. Return the roulade to the oven for 5 minutes.

Cole-slaw

Serves 4

6 oz (170g) white cabbage, shredded
2 medium carrots, grated
2 sticks celery, finely chopped
2–3 spring onions, chopped (optional)
3 tablespoons (45ml) reduced-calorie mayonnaise

1. Place all the vegetables in a large bowl. Add the mayonnaise and mix well.
2. Chill before serving.

Total CHO Neg

Total Cals 170

Stir-fried Vegetables

Serves 4–6

2 tablespoons (30ml) corn or sunflower oil
6 spring onions, chopped
1 carrot, peeled and cut into strips
1 small red pepper, deseeded and cut into strips
4 oz (115g) baby corn
4 oz (115g) mangetout, topped and tailed
4 oz (115g) broccoli, cut into 1-inch (2.5cm) pieces
4 oz (115g) button mushrooms, sliced
1 tablespoon (15ml) soya sauce
1 tablespoon (15ml) oyster sauce

1. Heat the oil in the wok until smoking. Add the spring onions, carrot and pepper. Stir-fry for 1 minute.
2. Add the remaining vegetables and stir-fry for a further 1–2 minutes. Add the soya sauce and oyster sauce, tossing the vegetables to combine all the ingredients.
3. Cook for a further 1–2 minutes and serve immediately.

Total CHO 20g

Total Cals 400

Courgette and Sweet Corn Flan

Serves 3–4

For the pastry:

4 oz (115g) wholemeal flour
2 oz (55g) plain flour
2 oz (55g) low-fat spread
1 oz (30g) white vegetable fat

For the filling:

1 medium courgette, sliced
3 oz (85g) sweet corn
2 oz (55g) reduced-fat Cheddar cheese
2 size 3 eggs, beaten
¼ pint (140ml) skimmed milk

1. To make the pastry, rub the fat into the flour. Knead to a smooth dough with enough water to bind. Use to line an 8-inch (20cm) flan ring. Chill in the refrigerator for 15–20 minutes.
2. Bake blind at 400°F/200°C (Gas Mark 6) for 10 minutes.
3. Place the courgette, sweet corn and cheese in base of the flan case. Mix the eggs and milk. Pour over the vegetables.
4. Bake at 350°F/180°C (Gas Mark 4) for 35 minutes or until springy to the touch.

Total CHO 140g

Total Cals 1440

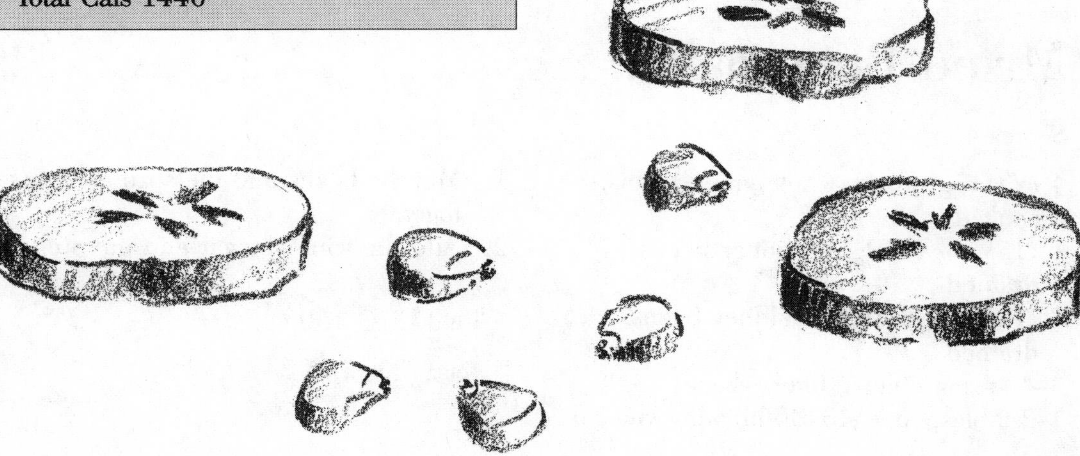

Leek Flan

Serves 6

For the pastry:

6 oz (170g) wholemeal flour
Pinch of salt
2 oz (55g) low-fat spread
1 oz (30g) white vegetable fat
Water to bind

For the filling:

1 onion, chopped
1 medium leek, thinly sliced
4 oz (115g) reduced-fat cheese
2 size 3 eggs, beaten
¼ pint (140ml) skimmed milk

1. To make the pastry, rub the fat into flour and salt. Knead to a smooth dough with sufficient water to bind. Line an 8-inch (20cm) flan ring.
2. Bake blind at 350°F/180°C (Gas Mark 4) for 10 minutes.
3. Arrange the onion and leek over the base. Sprinkle with cheese.
4. Pour over the egg and milk mixture. Bake at 350°F/180°C (Gas Mark 4) for 35 minutes or until firm to the touch.

Total CHO 120g

Total Cals 1350

Mixed Bean Salad

Serves 4–6

4 oz (115g) frozen whole green beans, cooked
1×15½ oz (439g) tin butter beans, drained
1×15½ oz (439g) tin kidney beans, drained
3–4 spring onions, finely sliced
1–2 tablespoons (15–30ml) wine vinegar

1. Mix the beans and the spring onions together.
2. Add the wine vinegar and mix well.

Total CHO 100g

Total Cals 530

Stir-fried Beansprouts

Serves 4

1 tablespoon (15ml) oil
1 clove garlic, crushed
1 red pepper, deseeded and cut into strips
6 spring onions, chopped
8 oz (225g) beansprouts
2 oz (55g) unsalted cashew nuts
2 tablespoons (30ml) soya sauce
1 tablespoon (15ml) red wine vinegar

Total CHO 10g

Total Cals 530

1. Heat the oil in a wok. Add the garlic, pepper and spring onions and stir-fry for 1 minute.
2. Add the beansprouts and nuts, mix well and cook for a further 1–2 minutes.
3. Add the soya sauce and wine vinegar, tossing well.

Artichokes with Tomatoes

Serves 4

1 lb (455g) Jerusalem artichokes
Sea salt and freshly ground black pepper
2 tablespoons (30ml) olive oil
1×14 oz (400g) tin tomatoes
1 teaspoon (5ml) dried marjoram *or* 1 tablespoon (15ml) fresh marjoram, chopped

Total CHO Neg

Total Cals 390

1. Cook artichokes in boiling, salted water for 20 minutes until tender. Drain and cut into even-sized pieces.
2. Meanwhile, heat the oil in another pan, add tomatoes, marjoram and artichokes. Season to taste.
3. Cover and simmer for 5–10 minutes until artichokes are soft and warmed through.
4. Transfer to a warmed dish. Serve immediately.

Bean and Cashew Nut Salad

Serves 4

1×15 oz (425g) cannellini beans, drained
2 sticks celery, finely chopped
1 red eating apple, cored and cut into cubes
3 spring onions, sliced
2 oz (55g) unsalted cashew nuts

For the dressing:

3 tablespoons (45ml) corn or sunflower oil
Juice of 1 lemon
1 tablespoon (15ml) white wine vinegar
1 tablespoon (15ml) dry sherry
½ teaspoon (2.5ml) dried oregano
1 teaspoon (5ml) whole grain mustard
Sea salt and freshly ground black pepper
Radicchio and/or frisée lettuce

1. Place the beans in a bowl and mix with remaining salad ingredients.
2. Place the dressing ingredients in a screw-top jar, shake well to blend, then pour over the ingredients in the bowl.
3. To serve, place the salad on a bed of radicchio and/or frisée lettuce.

Total CHO 60g

Total Cals 1030

LOW-CALORIE DISHES

Eating more calories than you use up in your daily activities can make you gain weight, because your body stores these extra calories as fat. If you have a weight problem, the best approach to it is to consult a dietitian who will provide you with a calorie-controlled diet which will include all the nutrients you need to keep healthy. Don't be tempted to try one of those 'miracle', very low-calorie diets which promise that you will lose a stone (14 pounds/6kg) in weight in two weeks — they have very little long-term benefit; and don't automatically assume that everything from the health food shop is low in calories. Carrot cake can be high in vegetable oil and raw brown sugar.

One way of watching your weight is obviously to cook food made from low-calorie ingredients and to choose cooking methods which do not add extra calories. Since fat is a concentrated source of calories, cutting down on fried and sautéed foods can help to reduce your calorie intake. A diet that is filling is easier to follow, so a high-fibre diet can be helpful in slimming. The recipes in this section have been compiled using the principles of healthy eating while keeping calories to a minimum but with absolutely no compromise on taste. Slimming need not be boring any more.

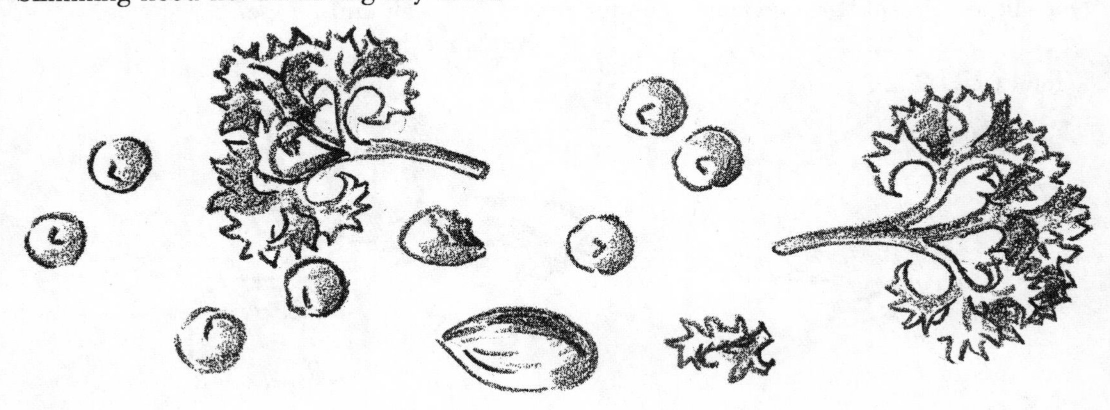

Carrots, Cabbage and Caraway

Serves 2

1 carrot, peeled and grated
½ small white or green cabbage, finely shredded
½ oz (15g) low-fat spread
1 tablespoon (15ml) caraway seeds
Sea salt and freshly ground black pepper

1. Place the vegetables in a steamer and cook for 10 minutes or until tender.
2. Toss the hot vegetables in the low-fat spread, caraway seeds and seasoning.
3. Serve immediately.

Total CHO Neg

Total Cals 80

Vegetable Medley

Serves 2

2 carrots, peeled and thinly sliced
1 leek, washed and sliced
1 small red pepper, diced coarsely
4 oz (115g) frozen sweet corn
Sea salt and freshly ground black pepper

1. Steam the carrots and leeks for 5 minutes.
2. Add the pepper and sweet corn and steam for a further 3 minutes. Toss with salt and pepper.
3. Serve hot.

Total CHO 20g

Total Cals 100

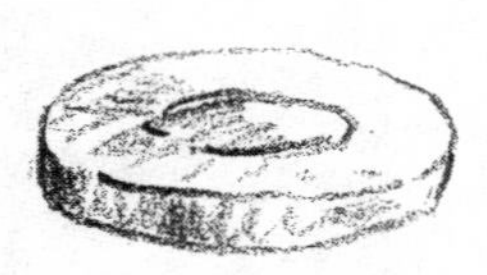

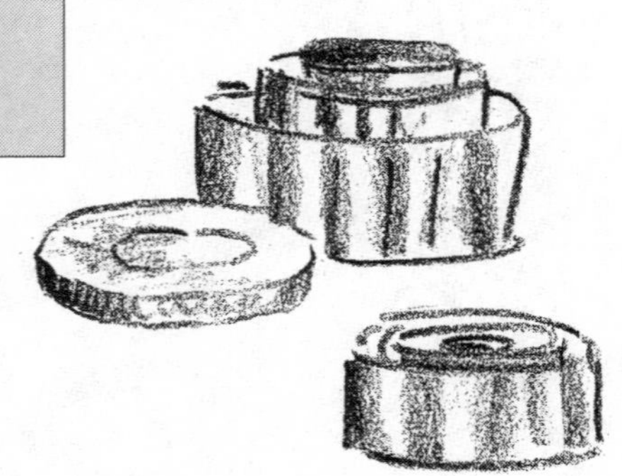

Beansprout Salad

Serves 4–6

1 green pepper, deseeded and sliced
1 small fennel, sliced
4 oz (115g) button mushrooms, sliced
2 sticks celery, sliced
4 oz (115g) beansprouts
1 oz (30g) alfalfa sprouts

1. Mix all ingredients together.
2. Toss with light vinaigrette dressing.

Total CHO Neg

Total Cals 80

Watercress Stuffed Tomatoes

Serves 4

4 large marmande or beefsteak tomatoes
1 bunch watercress, stalks removed and finely chopped
6 oz (170g) low-fat soft cheese
3 spring onions, finely chopped
1 teaspoon (5ml) creamed horseradish sauce
1 tablespoon (15ml) All-Bran
Sea salt and freshly ground black pepper to taste
A few spring onion curls

Total CHO Neg

Total Cals 350

1. Cut the stalk ends off the tomatoes, scoop out and discard the flesh.
2. Mix the watercress into the cheese with the spring onions, creamed horseradish, All-Bran and seasoning.
3. Pile into the tomato shells. Chill in refrigerator.
4. Before serving, garnish with spring onion curls* and salad.

*For spring onion curls, see page 101.

Chicken Salad

Serves 4–6

8 oz (225g) cooked chicken, diced
3 oz (85g) brown rice, cooked
3 oz (85g) reduced-fat Cheddar cheese, cubed
2 red eating apples, diced (reserve 3–4 slices)
2 oz (55g) radishes, sliced
2 sticks celery, sliced
1×5 fl oz (150g) carton low-fat natural yogurt
1 tablespoon (15ml) reduced-calorie mayonnaise

1. Mix the chicken, rice, cheese, apples, radishes and celery.
2. Combine the yogurt and mayonnaise and fold into the salad mixture. Garnish with the reserved apple slices.
3. Chill before serving.

Total CHO 100g

Total Cals 1100

Mediterranean Cod

Serves 4

4×4 oz (115g) cod steaks
2 teaspoons (10ml) lemon juice
Sea salt and freshly ground black pepper
1 oz (30g) low-fat spread
1 small onion, chopped
1 small pepper, chopped
1 stick celery, finely chopped
1×8 oz (225g) tin tomatoes, chopped
½ teaspoon (2.5ml) basil or oregano

Total CHO Neg

Total Cals 440

1. Place the fish in an ovenproof dish. Sprinkle with lemon juice and seasoning. Cook at 350°F/180°C (Gas Mark 4) for 15 minutes.
2. Meanwhile, gently melt the low-fat spread and sauté the onion, pepper and celery for 2–3 minutes.
3. Add the tomatoes and herbs, and season to taste. Spoon over the fish and cook for a further 15 minutes.

Vegetable Kebabs

Serves 4

For the marinade:

2 tablespoons (30ml) oil
1 tablespoon (15ml) fresh parsley, finely chopped
1 small onion, finely chopped
1 clove garlic, finely chopped
Sea salt and freshly ground black pepper

For the kebab:

1 red pepper, deseeded and cut into cubes
1 green pepper, deseeded and cut into cubes
2 courgettes, sliced
12 button mushrooms

1. Combine all the marinade ingredients, mixing well. Add the vegetables and coat thoroughly. Cover and leave in the refrigerator for approximately 2 hours.
2. Mix again. Thread the vegetables alternately onto skewers.
3. Grill for about 20 minutes, turning frequently, until tender.

Total CHO Neg

Total Cals 360

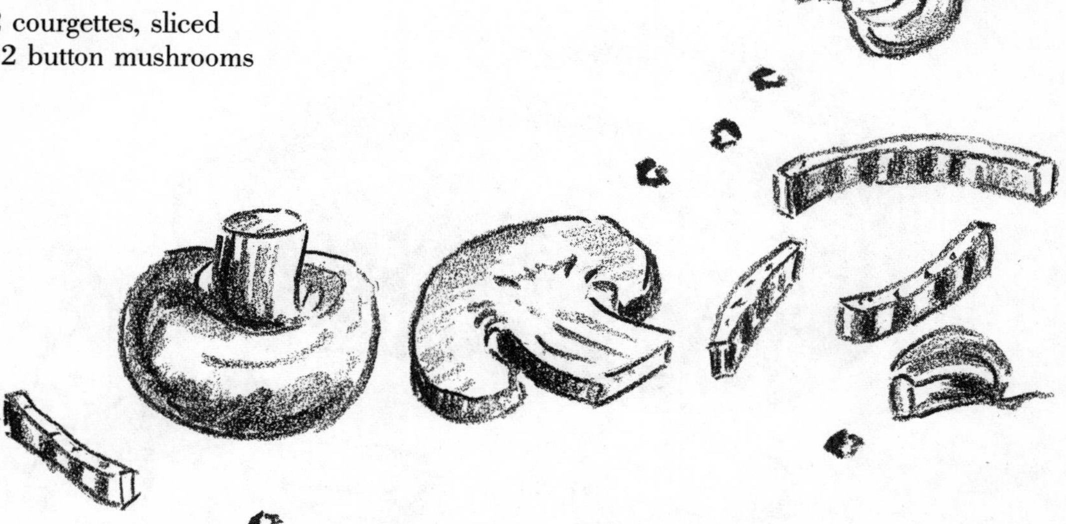

Ratatouille

Serves 4–6

1 aubergine, sliced
2 tablespoons (30ml) corn oil
1 onion, sliced
1 clove garlic, crushed
3 courgettes, sliced
1 green pepper, deseeded and sliced
1 red pepper, deseeded and sliced
1×14 oz (400g) tin tomatoes
1 tablespoon (15ml) tomato purée
Freshly ground black pepper

Total CHO Neg

Total Cals 300

1. Sprinkle the aubergine slices with salt and leave to stand for 30 minutes to remove bitter juices.
2. Meanwhile, heat the oil in a large pan. Add the onion and garlic and fry until golden. Add the remaining vegetables including the aubergines, season well with black pepper and stir in enough water to come about halfway up the mixture.
3. Bring to the boil, stirring constantly, then lower the heat, and simmer for approximately 30 minutes.
4. Adjust seasoning. Serve hot or cold.

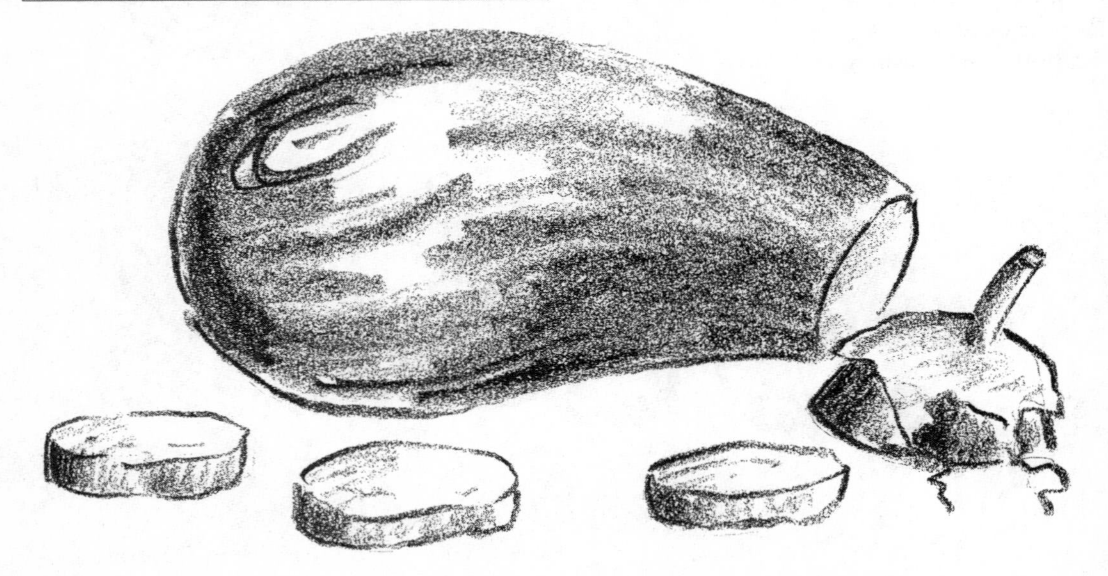

Plaice Provençal

Serves 4

4 skinned plaice fillets
½ lemon, sliced
½ oz (15g) low-fat spread

For the sauce:

1×14 oz (400g) tin tomatoes
1 clove garlic, crushed
1 small green pepper, finely chopped
1 small onion, finely chopped
1 teaspoon (5ml) provencal herbs
1 teaspoon (5ml) parsley, chopped
Sea salt and freshly ground black pepper

Total CHO Neg

Total Cals 350

1. Wash the fish and roll up each fillet neatly. Place in a medium gratin dish with slices of lemon in between. Dot with low-fat spread and cover with foil. Bake at 350°F/180°C (Gas Mark 4) for 10–12 minutes until the flesh is opaque.
2. Meanwhile, to make sauce, cook the tomatoes, garlic, pepper, onion, herbs, and parsley for 15–20 minutes until all the vegetables are soft and sauce reduced to a thick consistency. Stir occasionally to break up tomatoes.
3. Transfer the fish to a serving dish and pour over the sauce.
4. Serve immediately.

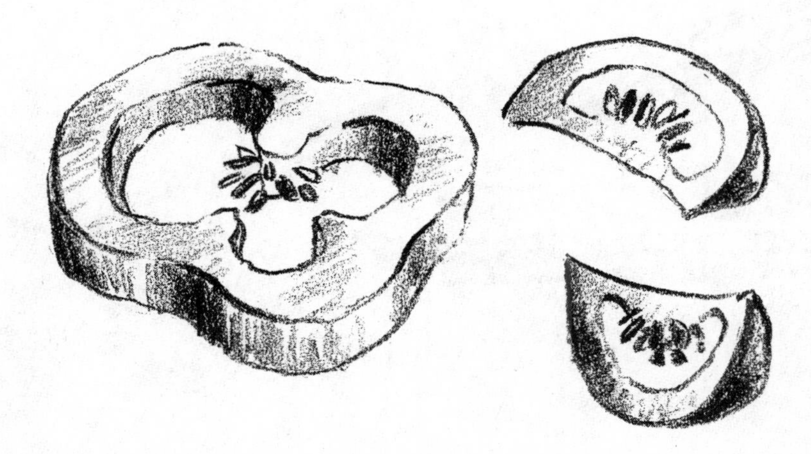

Greek Feta Salad

Serves 4–6

1 small onion, peeled and sliced
½ cucumber, cut into 3-inch (8cm) lengths
4 marmande or beefsteak tomatoes, sliced
3 oz (85g) Feta cheese, drained and sliced
2 oz (55g) black olives
2 tablespoons (30ml) olive oil
2 tablespoons (30ml) lemon juice
2 tablespoons (30ml) white wine vinegar
3 sprigs fresh mint, chopped
Sea salt and freshly ground black pepper

1. Arrange the onion, cucumber, tomato and Feta cheese on a serving plate. Add the olives.
2. Meanwhile, mix the oil, lemon juice and vinegar with the mint and seasoning. Shake dressing well and pour over salad.
3. Serve.

Total CHO Neg

Total Cals 500

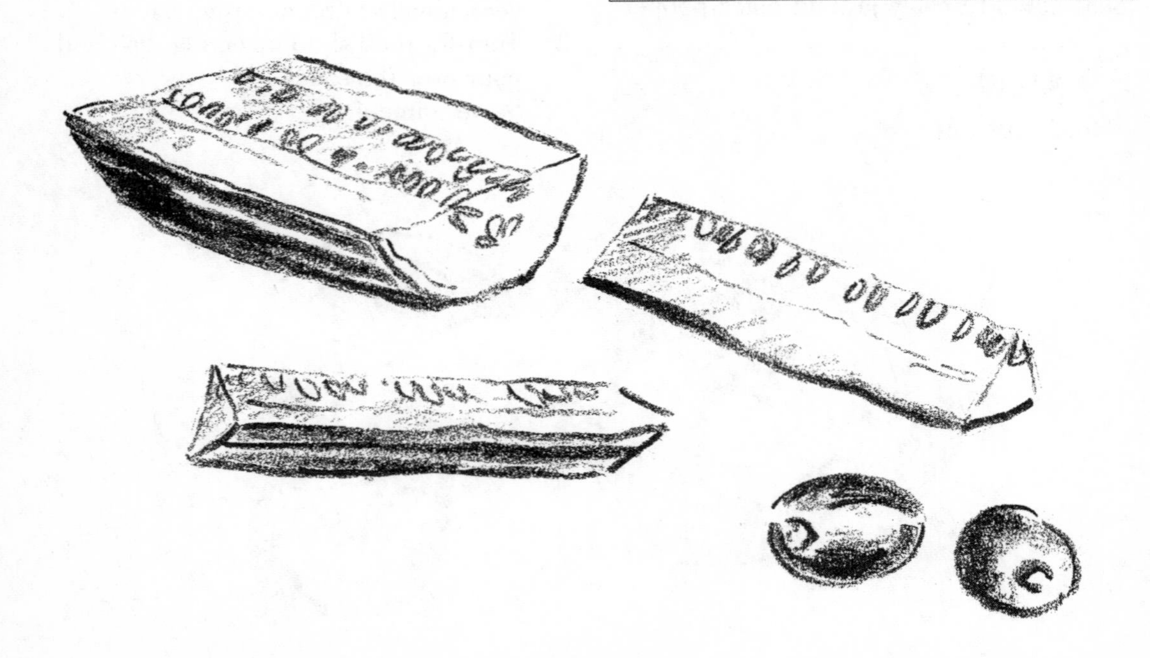

Salad Niçoise

Serves 4

1 lettuce, washed
4 tomatoes, quartered
8 oz (225g) fresh or frozen French beans
7 oz (200g) tin tuna in brine, drained and flaked
1 medium potato, cooked and cubed
1 small onion, sliced into rings
2 hard-boiled eggs, quartered
12 black olives
Lettuce leaves

For the dressing:

1 tablespoon (15ml) white wine or cider vinegar
3 tablespoons (45ml) olive oil
Pinch of dry mustard
Sea salt and freshly ground black pepper

1. Arrange the lettuce in a bowl. Add the tomatoes, beans, fish and potatoes.
2. Reserve a few onion rings and black olives for decoration and add the remainder to the bowl.
3. Mix the vinegar, oil, mustard, salt and pepper together to make the dressing. Pour over salad ingredients. Toss well and serve on a bed of lettuce leaves.
4. Garnish with the remaining onion rings and olives. Serve at once.

Total CHO 40g

Total Cals 780

SAUCES AND DRESSINGS

These accompaniments are designed to enhance the flavour of a dish and to add moisture to dry foods. However, they can be high in fat because they are often made from cream or oil. Skimmed milk and low-fat spread can reduce the fat content of an otherwise rich sauce without compromising on flavour. Basing salad dressings on vinegar, low-fat natural yogurt, lemon juice, or a purchased reduced-calorie mayonnaise can do the same thing for that tossed crisp salad.

Light Vinaigrette Dressing

Serves 4

3 tablespoons (45ml) sunflower oil
1 tablespoon (15ml) tarragon wine vinegar
½ teaspoon (2.5ml) English mustard powder
Sea salt and freshly ground black pepper

1. Place all ingredients in a screw-top jar with 1 tablespoon (15ml) water.
2. Shake well.

Total CHO Neg

Total Cals 400

French Dressing

Serves 4–6

4 tablespoons (60ml) sunflower oil
2 tablespoons (30ml) vinegar
Sea salt and freshly ground black pepper
Pinch of dry mustard

1. Place all ingredients in a jar with a screw-top lid.
2. Shake well.

Total CHO Neg

Total Cals 540

Mayonnaise

Serves 4

1 egg
¼ teaspoon (1.25ml) French mustard
2 tablespoons (30ml) wine vinegar
½ pint (285ml) sunflower oil

Total CHO Neg

Total Cals 2470

1. Bring the mustard, vinegar and oil to room temperature.
2. Place the egg, mustard, seasoning and 1 tablespoon (15ml) vinegar in a blender. Cover and run at maximum speed.
3. Pour in half the oil *very slowly*.
4. Stop motor, add remaining oil.
5. Switch on to maximum speed and pour in remaining vinegar until all is mixed in.

Piquant Dressing

Serves 4

1×5 fl oz (150g) carton low-fat natural yogurt
1 clove garlic, crushed
Pinch dry mustard
2 teaspoons (10ml) Worcestershire sauce
2–3 drops Tabasco sauce

1. Stir all ingredients into the yogurt and mix well.
2. Chill before serving.

Total CHO 10g

Total Cals 80

Raita

Serves 4–6

2×5 fl oz (150g) cartons low-fat natural yogurt
1 clove garlic, crushed
1 teaspoon (5ml) ground cumin
Sea salt and freshly ground black pepper
1 green chilli, seeded and chopped
Coriander leaves

1. In a bowl mix the yogurt, garlic, cumin, salt and pepper.
2. Sprinkle with the chilli and coriander leaves.

Total CHO 20g

Total Cals 160

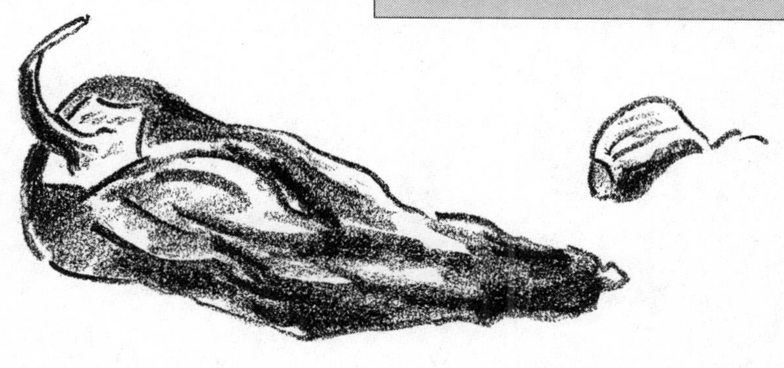

Tzatziki

Serves 4–6

2×5 fl oz (150g) cartons low-fat natural yogurt
4-inch (10cm) piece cucumber, diced
1 tablespoon (15ml) fresh mint, chopped
1 clove garlic, crushed (optional)
1 sprig fresh mint for garnish

1. Mix together all the ingredients.
2. Chill before serving garnished with the sprig of mint.

Total CHO 20g

Total Cals 180

PUDDINGS AND DESSERTS

It is often assumed that the only virtuous way to end a meal is with fresh fruit or a yogurt. Although these can be very refreshing, they can also be a little dull — your dinner party deserves a more exciting finale. By cutting down on the amount of sugar, and by using wholemeal flour, nuts, dried fruits, low-fat spread, and artificial intense sweeteners, you can once again enjoy a choice of hot and cold puddings.

Stripey Fool

Serves 6

10 oz (285g) raspberries or blackcurrants puréed (reserve 6)
½ pint (285ml) skimmed milk
2 tablespoons (30ml) cornflour
2 size 3 egg yolks
3–4 drops vanilla essence
Intense sweetener to taste
¼ pint (140ml) whipping cream, whipped

Total CHO 50g

Total Cals 930

1. Mix a little milk with cornflour and egg yolks. Heat the remaining milk until boiling and add to the cornflour. Stir well and pour back into the pan.
2. Stir continuously until thick. Add vanilla essence and sweeten to taste.
3. Cool. Fold in whipped cream.
4. Spoon layers of custard and fruit purée into a glass bowl or individual wine glasses. Top with a swirl of custard and decorate with the reserved fruit.
5. Chill before serving.

Apple and Mincemeat Jalousie

Serves 12

1×12 oz (340g) packet wholemeal puff pastry
2 cooking apples, stewed
2 tablespoons (30ml) mincemeat
2 teaspoons (10ml) lemon juice
Powdered intense sweetener, to taste
2 teaspoons (10ml) skimmed milk
1 egg white, to glaze

Total CHO 180g
Total Cals 1480

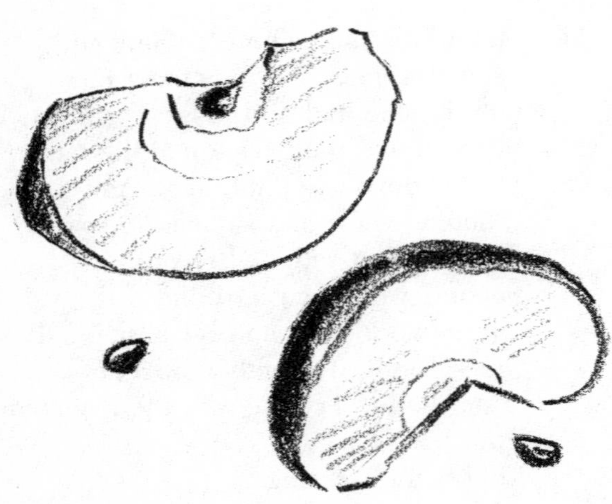

1. Cut the pastry in half. Roll out one half to approximately 14 in.×8 in. (35cm×20cm), and place on a greased baking tray.
2. Add the mincemeat to the apple and lemon juice and sweeten to taste. Spread this mixture over the pastry base, leaving ½-inch (1cm) border around the edge. Brush the edges with the milk.
3. Roll out remaining pastry to same size. Fold in half and cut slits from the fold to the outer edge, leaving a border around the edges. Place on top of apple and unfold to cover the apple completely. Seal the edges.
4. Glaze with lightly beaten egg white. Bake at 450°F/230°C (Gas Mark 8) for 15 minutes or until pastry is cooked.
5. As it comes out of the oven sprinkle with 1–2 tablespoons (15–30ml) powdered intense sweetener.

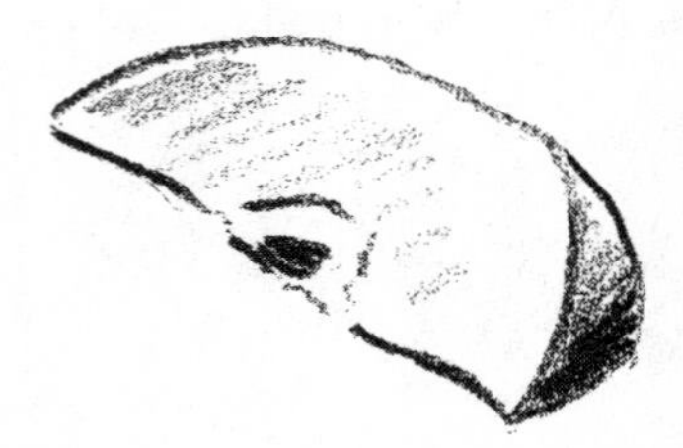

Apricot Creams

Serves 6

1×14 oz (411g) tin apricots in natural juice, drained and juice reserved
2×3 oz (80g) pots apricot fromage frais
1 size 3 egg, separated
1 teaspoon (5ml) lemon juice
1×½ oz (11g) sachet gelatine

Total CHO 60g
Total Cals 340

1. Strain the juice from the apricots into a basin. Add the lemon juice and sprinkle over the gelatine. Dissolve the gelatine by standing the bowl in a saucepan, half-filled with gently simmering water.
2. Purée the apricots in a liquidizer or blender. Stir the fruit purée and fromage frais into the dissolved gelatine. Sweeten to taste.
3. Whisk the egg white until stiff, then gently fold into the mixture.
4. Pour into one dish or 6 individual dishes. Allow to set in the refrigerator.

Kiwi and Lemon Syllabub

Serves 4–6

4 kiwi fruit
1×5 fl oz (150g) carton whipping cream
3 tablespoons (45ml) medium dry white wine
Zest and juice of ½ lemon
Intense sweetener to taste

Total CHO 20g
Total Cals 700

1. Peel the kiwi fruit and slice enough to line 4–6 goblets or wine glasses. Chop the rest and place in the base of the glasses.
2. Whisk the cream, wine and lemon juice until thick and floppy. Sweeten to taste.
3. Spoon into glasses. Chill for ½ hour in refrigerator. Serve.

Mango Fool

Serves 4

1 mango
3 teaspoons (15ml) orange liqueur
1×5 oz (150g) carton low-fat natural yogurt
1 orange, segmented and juice reserved

Total CHO 40g

Total Cals 280

1. Remove the flesh from the mango and purée with orange liqueur. Fold in the yogurt and orange juice.
2. Reserve 4 orange segments and divide the remaining pieces between individual serving dishes.
3. Pour in the mango purée and garnish with remaining orange segments. Chill before serving.

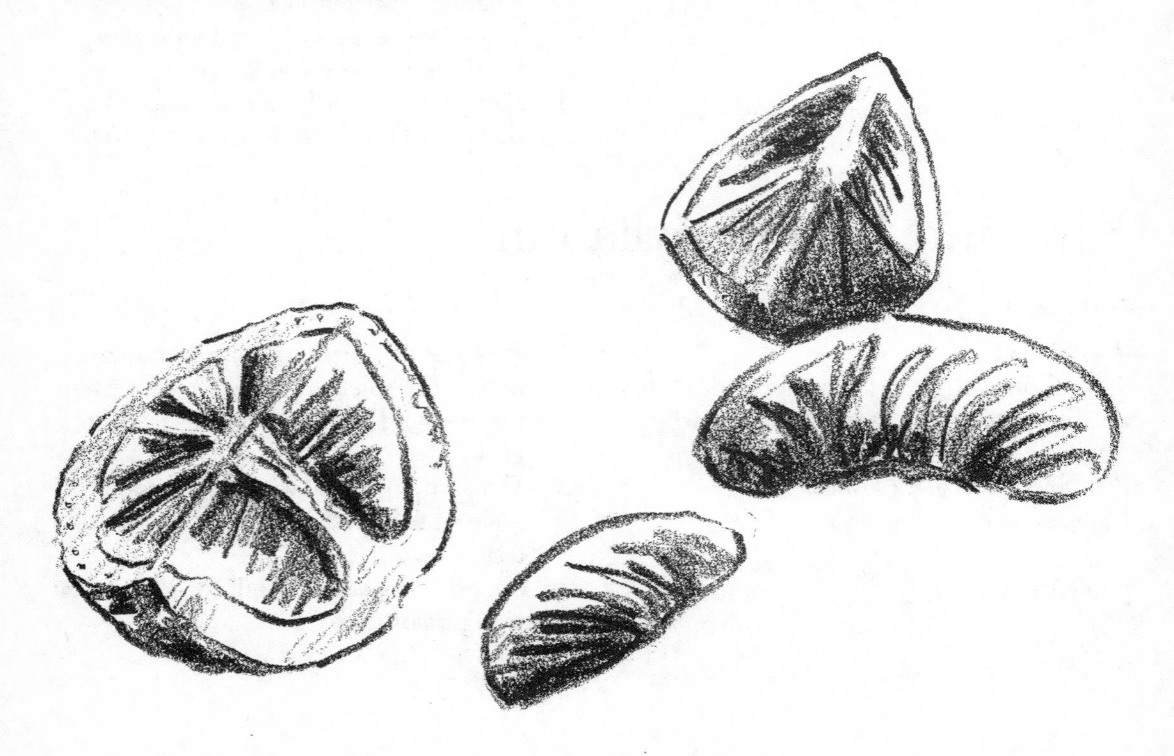

Summer Pudding

Serves 6

1½ lb (680g) mixed soft fruits (blackcurrants, redcurrants, raspberries or blackberries)
Intense sweetener to taste
6–8 slices stale white bread, crusts removed

Total CHO 130g

Total Cals 650

1. Place the soft fruits in a saucepan and cook gently for 5 minutes or until the juices run and the fruits soften. Sweeten to taste.
2. Meanwhile, line the base and sides of a 1½ pint (850ml) pudding basin with the bread, ensuring there are no gaps between the slices. Reserve 1½ slices for the top.
3. Put the fruit and all but 2 tablespoons (30ml) of the juice into the bread-lined basin. Cover with the reserved bread, put a plate over the top and weigh down. Chill overnight.
4. To unmould, invert a serving plate over the bowl and turn the pudding over. Use the reserved fruit juice to pour over any parts of the bread that have not been coloured.

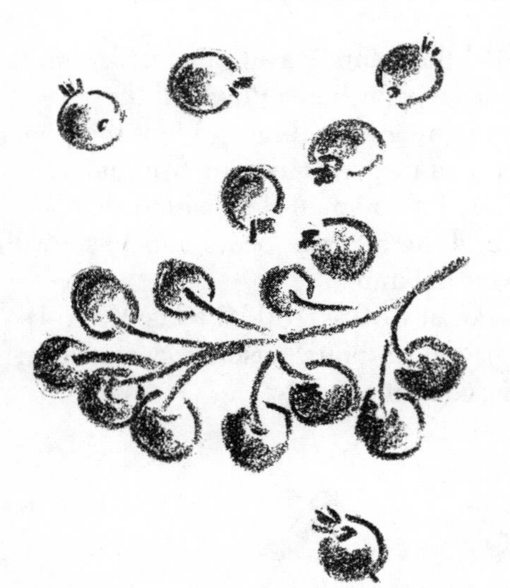

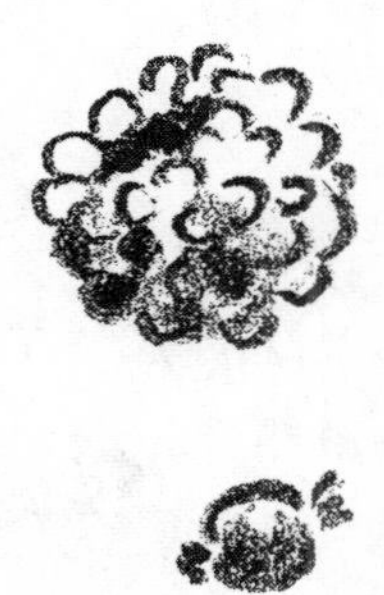

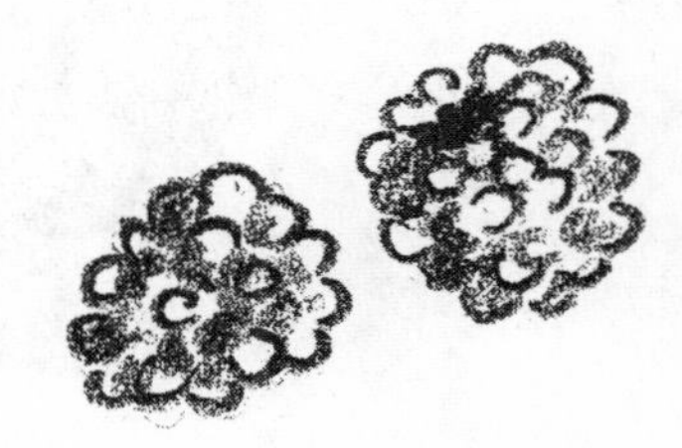

Pears in Mulled Wine

Serves 4

4 ripe, even-sized pears
½ pint (285ml) red wine
Pinch grated nutmeg
1 stick cinnamon
Rind of ½ lemon
A few drops lemon juice
4 cloves
A few drops intense sweetener to taste

Total CHO 40g
Total Cals 320

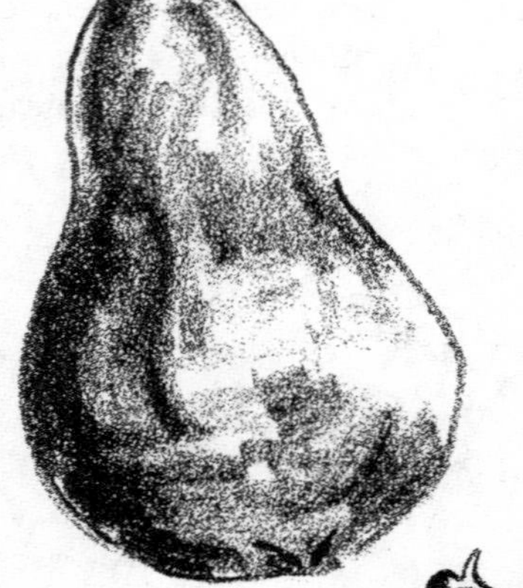

For a quick microwave method:

1. Peel pears leaving stalks on. Cut an even base. Place the remaining ingredients in a dish and cook in microwave for 5 minutes on full power.
2. Carefully place pears in wine, baste and return to microwave for 5 minutes on full power, stopping to baste at least once.
3. Leave to stand for 5 minutes; before serving baste the pears with the liquid.

For a conventional method:

1. Peel the pears leaving the stalks on. Cut an even base. Place all the remaining ingredients except the pears in a saucepan. Heat for 5 minutes.
2. Pour into a small deep-sided dish. Carefully add the pears and baste with wine mixture.
3. Bake at 350°F/180°C (Gas Mark 4) for half an hour, basting occasionally.
4. Serve immediately.

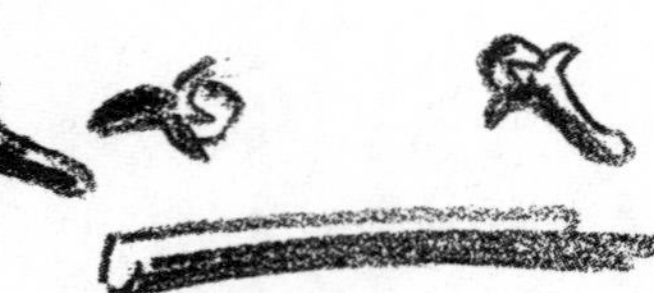

Cheesecake

Serves 6–8

2 oz (55g) low-fat margarine
6 oz (170g) wholemeal shortbread, crushed
1×½ oz (11g) sachet gelatine
Finely grated rind and juice of 1 orange
8 oz (225g) skimmed-milk cheese or quark
1×5 oz (150g) carton low-fat natural yogurt
Liquid-sweetener to taste, approx. 8 drops
2 size 3 eggs, separated
4 oz (115g) raspberries, fresh or frozen

Total CHO 100g

Total Cals 1465

1. Melt the margarine and mix in the crushed shortbread. Press down in an even layer in the base of a lightly greased 7-inch (18cm) spring-release tin or a loose-bottomed tart tin.
2. Chill in the refrigerator for 30 minutes.
3. Dissolve the gelatine in 3 tablespoons (45ml) hot water.
4. Put the orange rind and juice and skimmed-milk cheese into a bowl. Add the yogurt and egg yolks, and mix well together. Sweeten to taste. Add the cooled gelatine.
5. Whisk the egg whites until stiff and then lightly fold into the mixture. Carefully pour into the tin and chill for several hours.
6. Remove the cheesecake from the tin and place on a flat serving plate. Decorate with the fruit.

Cranberry Cheesecake

Serves 6–8

2 oz (55g) low-fat spread, melted
6 oz (170g) wholemeal shortbread, crushed
1×½ oz (11g) sachet gelatine, dissolved in 3 tablespoons (45ml) water
8 oz (225g) skimmed-milk cheese or quark
1×5 oz (150g) carton low-fat natural (plain) yogurt
1 size 3 egg, separated
5 oz (140g) cranberry sauce
Cream to decorate

Total CHO 150g
Total Cals 1500

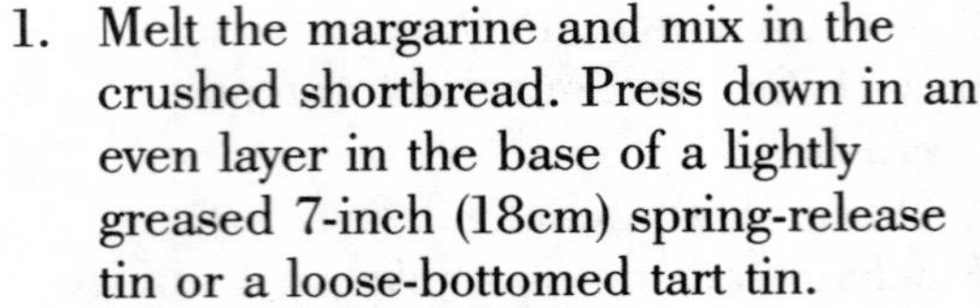

1. Melt the margarine and mix in the crushed shortbread. Press down in an even layer in the base of a lightly greased 7-inch (18cm) spring-release tin or a loose-bottomed tart tin.
2. Chill in the refrigerator for 30 minutes.
3. Dissolve the gelatine in 3 tablespoons (45ml) hot water. Put the skimmed-milk cheese, yogurt, egg yolk, and cranberry sauce in a large bowl and mix well together. Add the cooled gelatine.
4. Whisk the egg white until stiff and lightly fold into the mixture. Carefully pour the mixture on top of the crumb base and leave in the refrigerator until set.
5. Remove the cheesecake from the tin and place on a serving dish. Decorate with small rosettes of whipped cream and fresh cranberries if available.

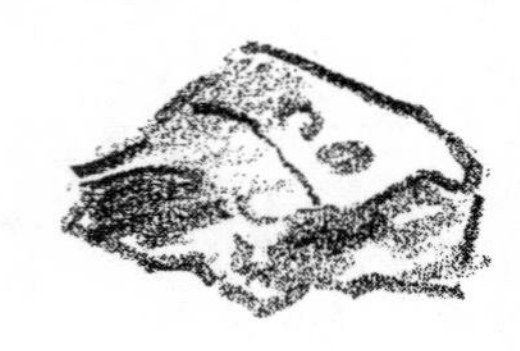

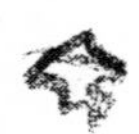

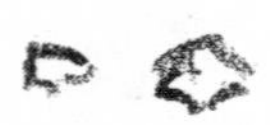

Tangy Fruits

Serves 4

4 oranges, peeled and segmented
8 oz (225g) fresh lychees, peeled and cut in half

1. Mix the fruits.
2. Chill well before serving.

Total CHO 60g

Total Cals 270

Tropical Pineapple Boats

Serves 6

1 medium pineapple, cut in half lengthways
1 mango
1 medium orange, peeled and segmented
2 passion fruit
2 kiwi fruit, peeled and sliced
Small bunch grapes, cut in half and pips removed

1. Scoop out the pineapple flesh from the skins and place in a bowl. Add the remaining fruits, reserving two slices of kiwi fruit, and mix well.
2. Fill the pineapple skins with the fruit.
3. Decorate with the sliced kiwi fruit.

Total CHO 100g

Total Cals 420

French Apple Flan

Serves 8–10

For the pastry:

6 oz (170g) wholemeal flour
1½ oz (45g) low-fat spread
1½ oz (45g) white vegetable fat
2–3 tablespoons (45ml) cold water

For the filling:

2 medium cooking apples
Intense sweetener to taste
2 eating apples
1 oz (30g) apricot pure fruit spread

Total CHO 160g

Total Cals 1280

1. Make the pastry and line a 9-inch (23cm) flan ring and bake blind at 400°F/200°C (Gas Mark 6) for 10–15 minutes.
2. Meanwhile, peel and chop up cooking apples and stew for 5–8 minutes until apple is a soft pulp. Sweeten to taste. Spread this mixture over the cooked flan case.
3. Core the eating apples and cut into quarters, slice very thinly and arrange on top of the tart in concentric circles.
4. Gently heat the apricot purée, adding 1 tablespoon (15ml) water if necessary to make a runny consistency.
5. Brush over apples to glaze.

Fresh Fruit Jelly

Serves 8

1×½ oz (13g) sugar-free jelly crystals
1 red apple, cored and sliced
1 orange, peeled and segmented
20 grapes (10 black and 10 white)

Or:

Use any fresh fruit available, e.g. strawberry, banana, tangerines.

1. Make up jelly following the instructions on the packet. Layer the fruit in a 2-pint (1.1 litre) jelly mould.
2. Pour over the jelly and leave to set.

Total CHO 40g

Total Cals 170

AFTERNOON TEA

A light snack in the afternoon accompanied by a cup of tea can be a very welcoming gesture. Many people with diabetes feel that their diets will prevent them from eating cakes, scones or biscuits. However, it is perfectly possible to offer home-baked products which follow the dietary guidelines of a high-fibre, low-fat and low-sugar diet.

Raspberry Buns

Makes 18

4 oz (115g) wholemeal self-raising flour
4 oz (115g) self-raising flour
4 oz (115g) low-fat spread
2 oz (55g) granulated sugar
1 size 3 egg, beaten
⅛ pint (70ml) skimmed milk
3 tablespoons (45ml) pure fruit spread or sugar-free raspberry jam

Total CHO 250g

Total Cals 1575

1. Sieve the flour. Gently rub in the fat until it resembles fine breadcrumbs.
2. Add the sugar. Stir in the egg and milk and mix to a stiff dough.
3. Shape into buns and put ½ teaspoon (2.5ml) jam on top.
4. Bake at 400°F/200°C (Gas Mark 6) for 10–15 minutes.

Dundee Cake

Cuts into 16

6 oz (170g) low-fat spread
2 oz (55g) caster sugar
8 oz (225g) fine wholemeal self-raising flour
Pinch of salt
1 teaspoon (5ml) mixed spice
3 size 3 eggs, beaten
1 tablespoon (15ml) skimmed milk
7 oz (200g) mixed fruit
1 oz (30g) split almonds for decoration

Total CHO 335g

Total Cals 2550

1. Cream the low-fat spread and sugar until light and fluffy.
2. Add the eggs to the creamed mixture, one at a time, with a little of the flour. Stir, then beat thoroughly. Stir in the milk. Beat again.
3. Add the fruit and the rest of the flour, with salt and spice. Fold in lightly.
4. Place the mixture in a greased and lined 7-inch (18cm) round cake tin. Arrange the split almonds on top and bake at 350°F/180°C (Gas Mark 4) for an hour and at 300°F/150°C (Gas Mark 2) for a further 1–1¼ hours or until a skewer comes out clean.

Easy Fruit Cake

Cuts into 12

6 oz (170g) dried fruit
1 oz (30g) caster sugar
4 oz (115g) low-fat spread
½ pint (285ml) cold tea
1 size 3 egg
8 oz (225g) wholemeal self-raising flour
2 oz (55g) walnuts, chopped

Total CHO 300g

Total Cals 2100

1. Place the fruit, sugar, low-fat spread, and tea in a pan and simmer gently for 20 minutes. Cool slightly. Stir in the egg, flour and walnuts.
2. Place in a lined 6-inch (15cm) cake tin. Bake at 325°F/160°C (Gas Mark 3) for approximately 1½ hours or until a skewer comes out clean.
3. Cool in the tin.

Bran Fruit Loaf

Cuts into 20

4 oz (115g) All-Bran
2 oz (55g) caster sugar
6 oz (170g) dried mixed fruit
½ pint (285ml) tea
4 oz (115g) wholemeal self-raising flour

Total CHO 300g

Total Cals 1300

1. Put the All-Bran, sugar, fruit, and tea in a bowl, and mix well. Leave to stand for ½ hour. Stir in the flour.
2. Place in an oiled 2 lb (900g) loaf tin. Bake at 350°F/180°C (Gas Mark 4) for approximately one hour.
3. Allow to cool on a wire rack.

Note: This recipe freezes well wrapped in foil.

Raisin and Choc Chip Cookies

Makes approx. 30

4 oz (115g) low-fat spread
2 oz (55g) caster sugar
1 size 3 egg, beaten
½ teaspoon (2.5ml) vanilla essence
4 oz (115g) 81 per cent wholemeal flour
½ teaspoon (2.5ml) bicarbonate of soda
½ teaspoon (2.5ml) salt
2 oz (55g) plain chocolate, chopped
2 oz (55g) raisins

Total CHO 210g

Total Cals 1560

1. Cream the fat and sugar until light and fluffy. Beat in the egg and vanilla essence. Sieve the flour, bicarbonate of soda and salt and stir into the creamed mixture with the chocolate chips and raisins. Mix well.
2. Place teaspoonfuls evenly spaced onto a lightly greased baking sheet. Bake at 350°F/180°C (Gas Mark 4) for 12–15 minutes.
3. Allow to cool slightly on the baking sheet before transferring to a wire rack.

Coconut Biscuits

Makes 10–12

4 oz (115g) fine self-raising wholemeal flour
1 oz (30g) sugar
2 oz (55g) desiccated coconut
1 size 3 egg, beaten
2 oz (55g) low-fat spread, melted

Total CHO 110g

Total Cals 1130

1. Stir all the dry ingredients together. Add the beaten egg and low-fat spread and mix to a firm dough.
2. Shape into rounds and place on a lightly greased baking sheet. Bake at 350°F/180°C (Gas Mark 4) for 10–15 minutes.
3. Allow to cool on wire rack.

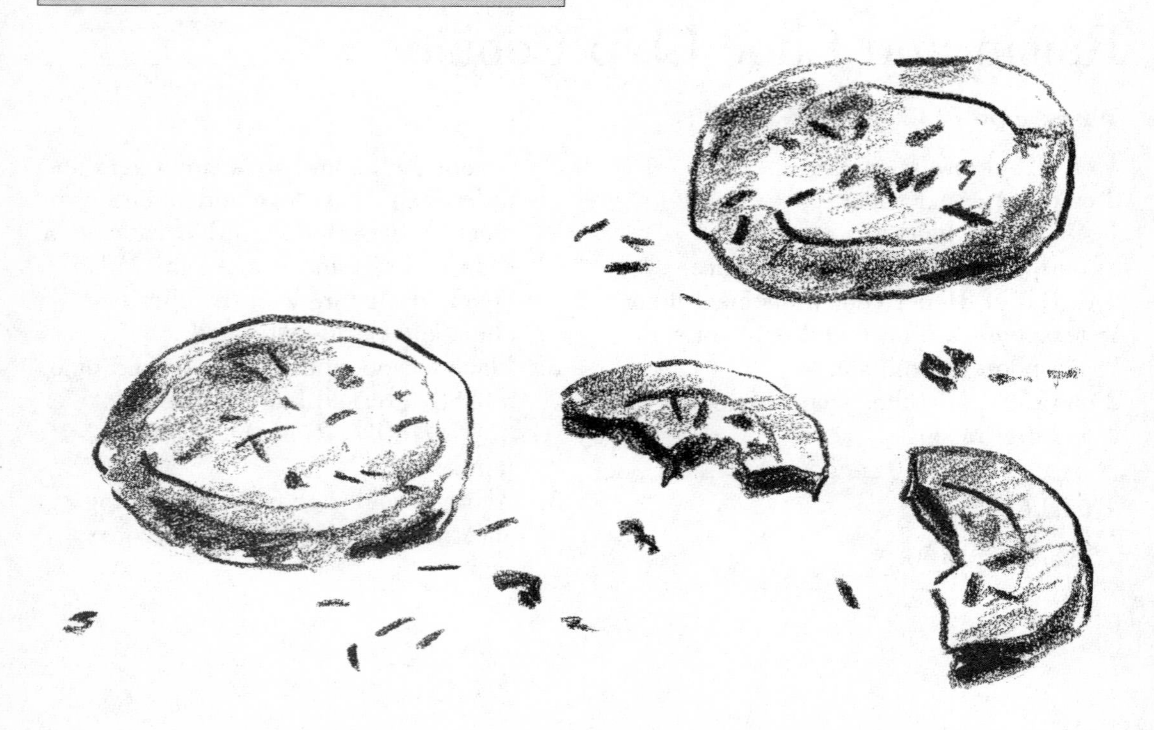

Wholemeal Fruit Flan

Serves 6–8

2 size 3 eggs
1 oz (30g) caster sugar
3 oz (85g) fine self-raising wholemeal flour
1 teaspoon (5ml) baking powder
1 tablespoon (15ml) warm water if necessary
Tinned fruit for filling
Arrowroot

Total CHO 90g*

Total Cals 550

1. Whisk the eggs and sugar together until thick and creamy. Sift the flour and baking powder (add back the bran left in the sieve) onto the mixture and quickly fold in using a metal spoon. Add the water if necessary.
2. Pour into a non-stick (or well-oiled) 7-inch (18cm) tin.Bake in the middle of a pre-heated oven at 400°F/200°C (Gas Mark 6) for approximately 8–10 minutes until brown, risen and firm. Turn out onto a cooling rack.
3. When completely cool, fill with fruit of choice, e.g. fruit cocktail in apple juice, mandarins in natural juice, etc.
4. Reserve a little of the juice and thicken slightly with a little arrowroot. Pour over the fruit and allow to set before serving.
5. Serve with a little single cream, evaporated milk or a small garnish of aerated cream.

* N.B. Remember to add on carbohydrate content of fruit of choice and arrowroot (1 tablespoon (15ml) = 10g CHO and 35 calories).

Melting Moments

Makes 12–14

3 oz (85g) fine self-raising wholemeal flour
2 oz (55g) self-raising flour
Pinch of salt
2½ oz (70g) white polyunsaturated vegetable fat
2½ oz (70g) low-fat spread
2 oz (55g) caster sugar
½ size 3 egg, beaten
Porridge oats
A few glacé cherries

Total CHO 185g

Total Cals 1740

1. Mix the flour and salt together. Cream the low-fat spread and vegetable fat, add the sugar, and cream again.
2. Beat in the egg and add a little flour. Stir in the rest of the flour.
3. Divide the mixture into 12–14 pieces. Roll each into a ball and toss in oats. Place on greased baking trays without flattening.
4. Decorate each Melting Moment with a piece of glacé cherry and bake at 350°F/180°C (Gas Mark 4) for 15 minutes.

FINISHING TOUCHES

To impress your guests, set aside a few extra minutes to make these simple garnishes. Some need chilling, so make them an hour or two in advance.

Spring onion curls

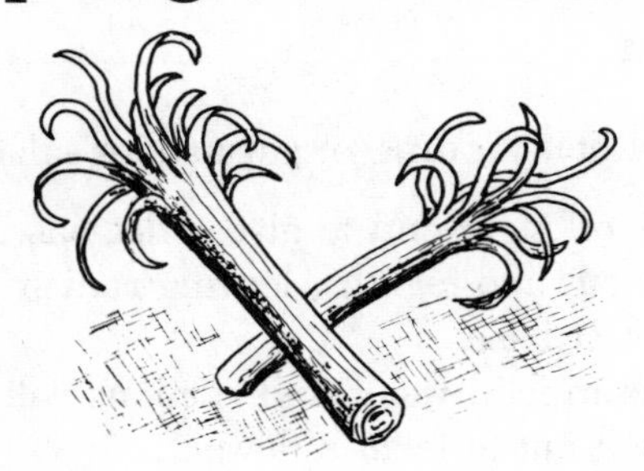

An impressive garnish for dips, cheeseboards and oriental dishes.

1. Trim the onions to 3 inches (7.5cm) in length, leaving a 1-inch (2.5cm) piece intact at bulb end. Finely slice stem lengthways.
2. Leave in iced water until ends curl. Drain.

Twists

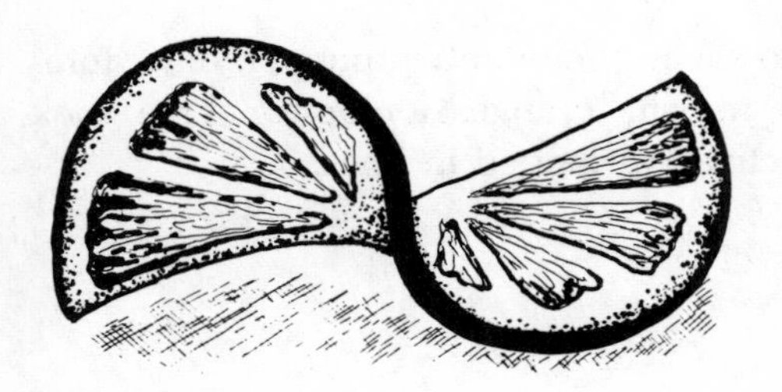

An ideal garnish for any fish dish or main meals served with a citrus sauce. Also suitable for chilled citrus desserts.

1. From the centre of a slice of lemon, orange or lime (also cucumber) make a cut to one edge.
2. Twist cut edges in opposite directions to form a curl. Try two slices together, e.g. lemon and lime for a colourful effect.

Gherkin fan

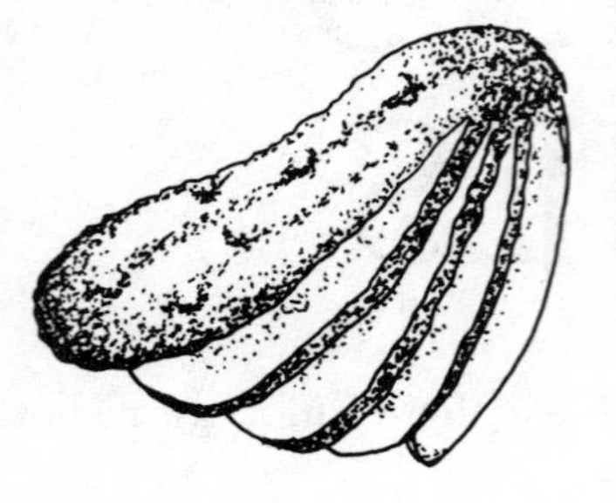

Ideal to garnish cheese dishes, open sandwiches and pâtés.

1. Slice gherkins lengthways, at equal intervals, leaving one end intact.
2. Gently spread these joined slices of gherkin apart to form a fan.

Radish waterlily

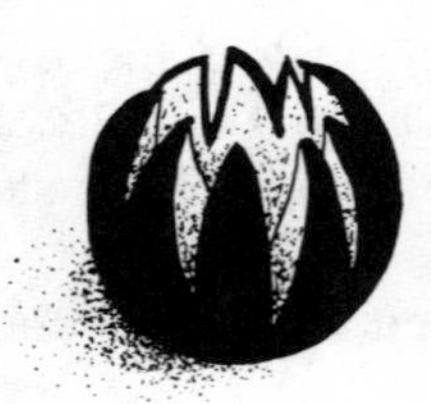

Ideal crudités for dips, or garnish for salads.

1. Slice off stem end to give a flat base, then cut into eighths, leaving radish intact at base.
2. Place in iced water and sections will spread out to form a flower.

Slices

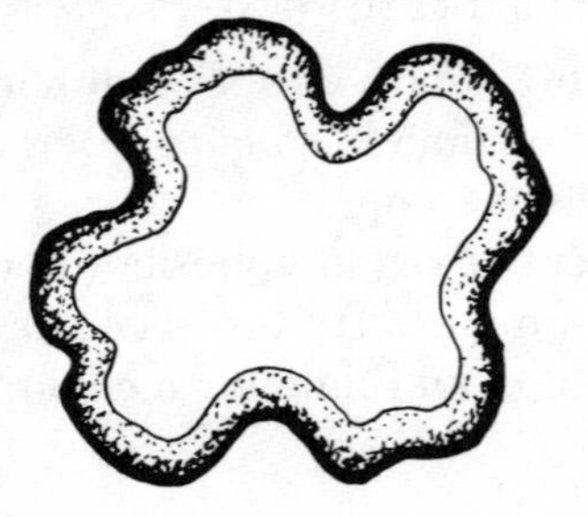

Thin slices of cucumber, pepper, olive, tomato, radish, orange, lemon or lime look effective overlapped in lines.

Celery curls

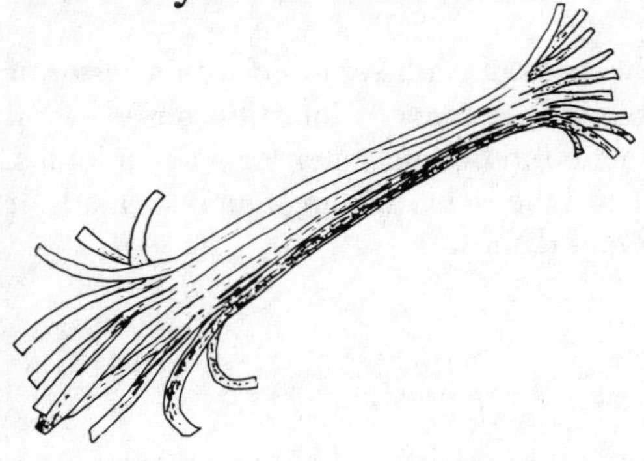

Ideal to garnish cheeseboards, open sandwiches, rice and noodle dishes.

1. Cut celery stalk into 2-inch (5cm) lengths and split in half lengthways. At each end make several lengthways cuts, leaving celery joined in the middle.
2. Chill in iced water. Drain.

Cut-outs

Use petal, flower or heart-shaped aspic cutters to cut tiny designs from peppers or citrus rinds. The shapes can be arranged to look like flowers.

Butterflies

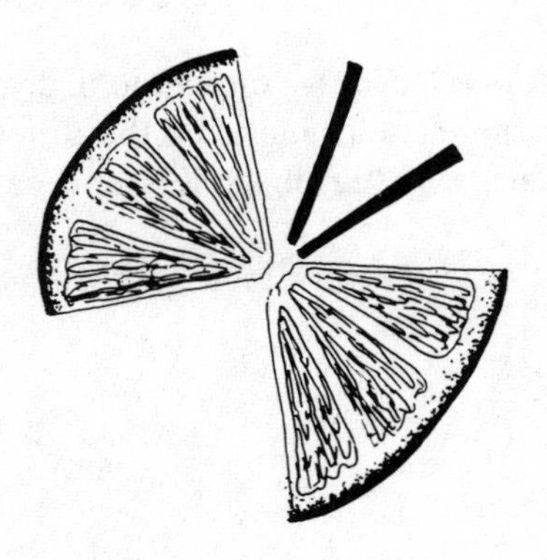

Cut a slice of lemon or orange into quarters and arrange two quarters in the shape of a butterfly. Add two tiny strips of pepper for antennae.

Citrus strips

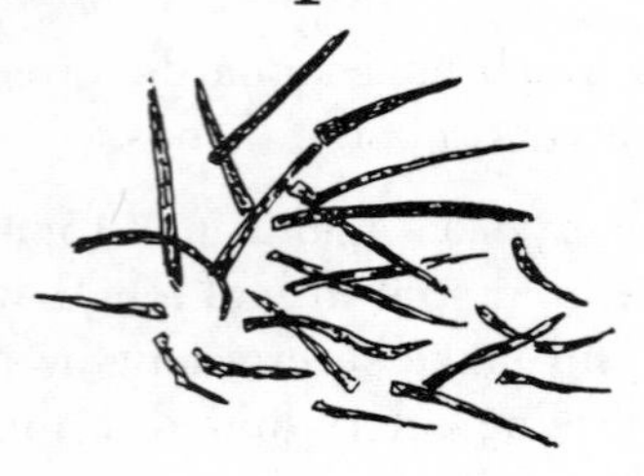

Thin strips of rind, removed with a zester or vegetable peeler, cut into thin shreds, and blanched in boiling water for a few minutes, can add the right finishing touch to salads or oriental dishes.

Lattice

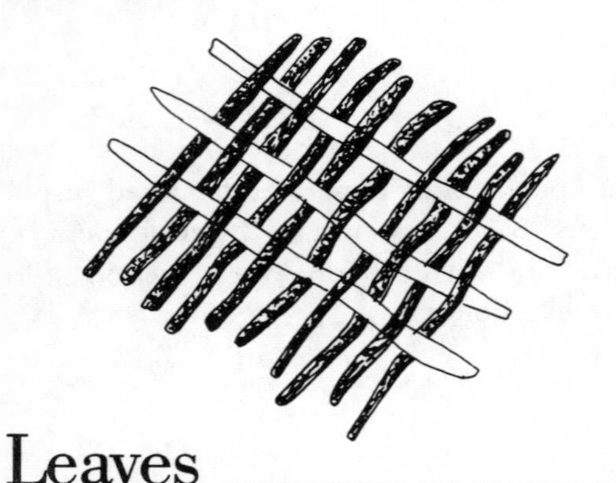

Arrange thin strips of pepper, spring onion, or anchovy fillets, halved lengthways, in a striking lattice design to decorate salads. (Anchovy fillets should first be soaked in milk for 20 minutes to remove excess salt.)

Leaves

Small lettuce leaves — radicchio, frilly lollo-rosso, frisée etc. can make all the difference to fish and egg starters, pâtés and savoury mousses.

Sprigs of watercress look good on soups.

Crimped slices

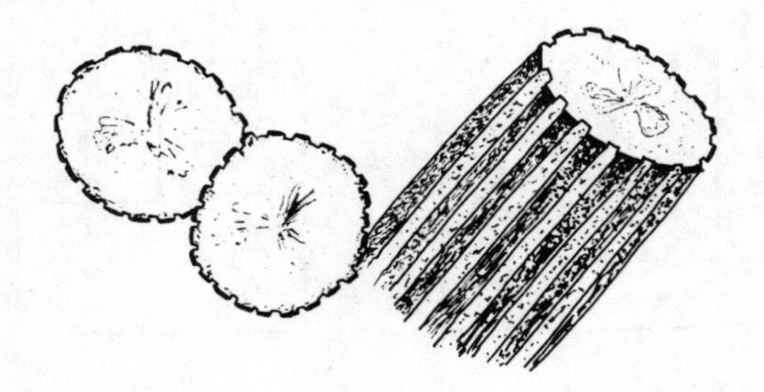

To garnish salads, pâtés, meat, fish or poultry dishes.

1. Use a canelle knife to remove narrow strips of skin or peel from cucumber, orange, lemon or lime. Discard the strips.
2. Cut the fruit or vegetable in slices.

Waterlily napkin

Open out napkin and lay flat in front of you (step 1).

Take each corner and fold into centre (step 2) until you have another square (step 3).

Take new corners and repeat. Repeat again. The napkin will now appear to be getting very small and you will have to hold all the points firmly in the middle.

Turn napkin over so that folds are face down, and bring corners into centre again, holding them firmly (step 4). From now on keep one hand holding the centre all the time.

Take each corner one by one and lift flap from underneath keeping the corner in shape to form a petal (steps 5a and 5b). Again take flaps from underneath but this time gently lay out to form another row of petals (step 6).

Now take out the final row of petals and pull each one tight this time, but make sure you are holding the centre firmly in place with the other hand (step 7).

The napkin is now ready to put on a plate (step 8).

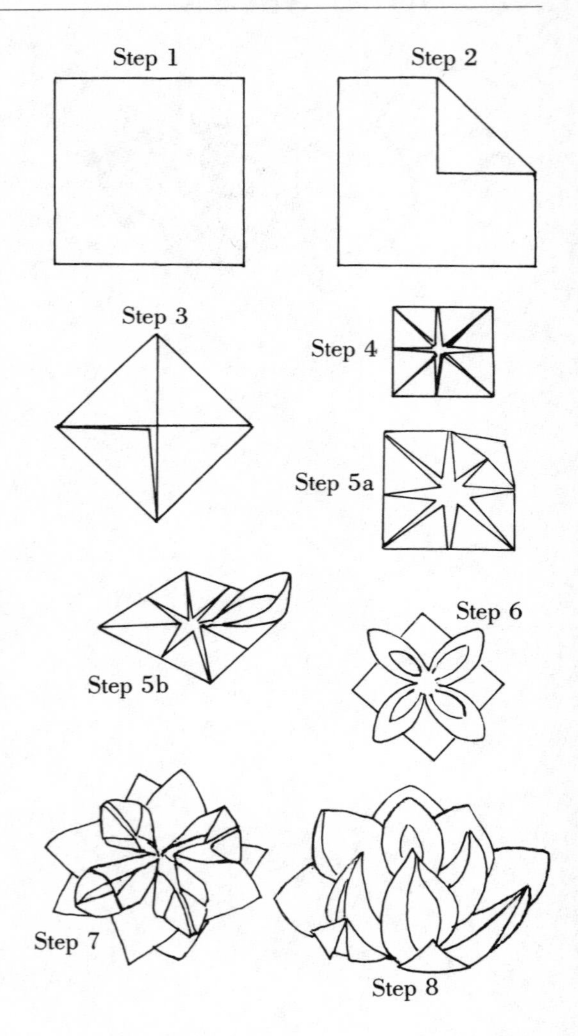

Bishop's mitre napkin

Lay napkin out flat in front of you (step 1).

Fold in half, straight side to straight side (step 2).

Take top right corner and fold down to centre of base fold (step 3).

Take bottom left corner and bring up to meet at the top (step 4).

Turn napkin over so that folds are face down (step 5).

Take top edge and fold down to meet bottom edge, leaving flaps loose (step 6).

Take bottom right corner and fold in under the flap on the left side (step 7), making sure that it fits right into the edge for a snug fit. Turn over (step 8).

Again take bottom right corner and fold in under the flap on the left side.

Now stand napkin up and gently shape into a round (step 9).

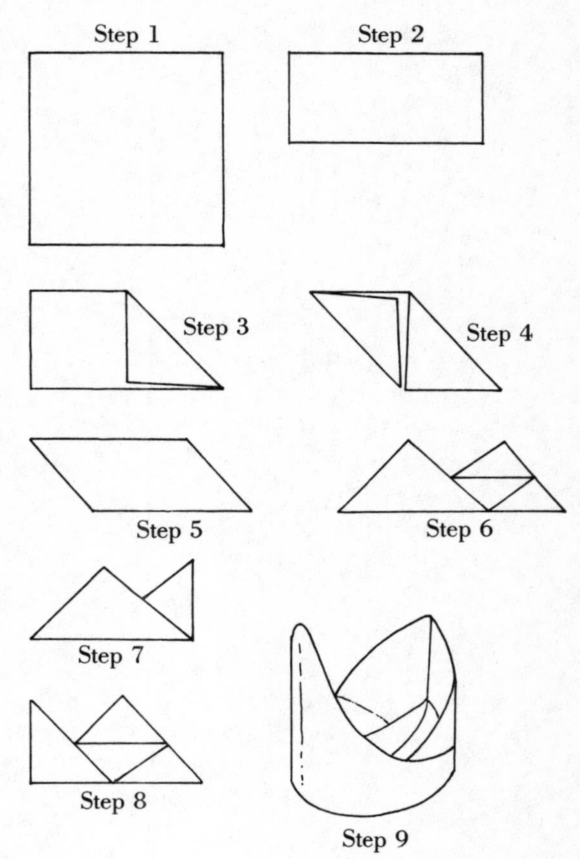

INDEX